Introduction to
Medical Office Transcription

Second Edition

Karonne J. Becklin

Edith M. Sunnarborg

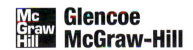

Glencoe
McGraw-Hill

New York, New York   Columbus, Ohio   Chicago, Illinois   Peoria, Illinois   Woodland Hills, California

Photo Credits

Courtesy of William H. Bush, Jr., M.D., University of Washington, Seattle 113; Corbis 39; Custom Medical Stock Photo, Inc. 53, 85, 145, 163; James Davis/International Stock 1; Tony Freeman/PhotoEdit 101; Image Bank 8; Lester Lefkowitz/Stock Market 69; Jose Luis Pelaez/Stock Market 129; Pictor 4, 9; Superstock 13; David Young Wolff/Stone 181

Library of Congress Cataloging-in-Publication Data

Becklin, Karonne J.
    Introduction to medical office transcription / Karonne J. Becklin, Edith M.
  Sunnarborg.--2nd ed.
        p. ; cm.
    Includes index.
    Rev. ed. of: Medical office transcription. c1998.
    ISBN 0-07-826260-7
    1. Medical transcription--Study and teaching (Higher) 2. Medical secretaries--Training
of. 3. Dictation (Office practice)--Problems, exercises, etc. 4. Allied health
personnel--Training of. I. Sunnarborg, Edith M. II. Becklin, Karonne J. Medical office
transcription. III. Title.
    [DNLM: 1. Medical Records--Problems and Exercises. 2. Medical
Records--Terminology--English. 3. Medical Secretaries. W 18.2 B397i 2003]
R28.8 .B42 2003
653'.18--dc21
                                                                            2001054316

Glencoe/McGraw-Hill

A Division of The McGraw·Hill Companies

Send all inquiries to:
Glencoe/McGraw-Hill
21600 Oxnard Street, Suite 500
Woodland Hills, CA 91367

ISBN 0-07-826260-7

1 2 3 4 5 6 7 8 9   079   06 05 04 03 02 01

Contents

Preface

Introduction to Medical Office Transcription, Second Edition, is designed for beginning medical transcription students. Many types of dictated medical documents, including chart notes, history and physical reports, consultations, office procedure notes, x-ray reports, progress notes, and letters, are provided.

The goals of the program are to develop transcribing speed and accuracy, gain skill in editing and proofing documents, and increase knowledge of medical terminology. Basic medical terminology, keyboarding, basic English skills, word processing basics, and general transcription skills are prerequisites for *Introduction to Medical Office Transcription*, Second Edition. Upon completion of the text-workbook and transcription, the student will

1. Apply written communication skills, including punctuation, capitalization, grammar, sentence structure, letter formats, report formats, and so forth.
2. Use designated references.
3. Review and apply medical terminology.
4. Maintain a medical word list.
5. Follow dictation instructions.
6. Apply basic medical transcription guidelines.
7. Develop speed during medical transcription.
8. Develop accuracy during medical transcription.
9. Transcribe and create appropriate medical documents.
10. Proof and edit medical documents.

To the Student

In using *Introduction to Medical Office Transcription*, Second Edition, you will work with this text-workbook and the accompanying dictation recordings. The program is divided into twelve chapters. Chapter 1 introduces the transcription process and provides information about a career in medical transcription, professionalism and the AAMT. This chapter also covers the work environment and work quality, a summary of basic medical transcription guidelines, and editing and proofing information. Chapter 2 introduces the patient medical record, types of medical documents and their formats, and reviews medical word building.

Chapters 3 through 11 begin with a short description of the anatomy and function of each body system. Common structures are labeled on appropriate diagrams, and key anatomical words are given in italics. Chapter 12 reviews previous chapters by providing case studies about several patients.

Structure of the Chapters

Following the introductory material in Chapters 1 and 2, Chapters 3 through 11 each cover a particular body system. These chapters present key concepts and terms that appear in the recorded dictation that you will transcribe. Chapters are organized as follows:

- **Objectives** A list of the major objectives covered in the chapter.
- **Anatomy** A short description of the anatomy and function of the system.
- **Clinical Assessment** An explanation of the observations made by the physician (examiner) when evaluating the system.
- **Symptoms and Disease Conditions** Terms that describe symptoms, signs, and names of disease conditions with pronunciation information and brief definitions. These terms are used in corresponding chapter transcription.
- **Medical and Surgical Procedures** Commonly performed procedures and laboratory tests.
- **Medications** A list of related medications with the pronunciation and classification of each drug.
- **Related Terms** Additional terms used in dictation for the chapter.
- **Editing and Proofing Guidelines** A review of the basic English skills necessary for transcribing the chapter's dictation.
- **Review** Exercises to test your understanding of the chapter.
- **Hints for Transcription** Transcribing points for the dictation.
- **Transcription Checkoff Sheet** List of transcription exercises that serves as a record of your progress. There are columns for you to enter each item's start and completion date, as well as the grade and/or number of errors on that item.

Organization of the Recordings

The dictation for each chapter begins with a recording of the symptom and disease condition terms that provides practice in word recognition and pronunciation. Listen and follow along in the text-workbook as each term is pronounced. You may wish to listen to the pronunciation a second time in order to practice spelling the terms.

The second part of each dictation provides the various medical reports and letters dictated for the chapter. Follow the text-workbook's instructions for the format of each document. Your instructor may provide additional guidelines concerning letterhead or formats for you to follow.

Content of the Appendices

The appendices provide references, drug classifications, common abbreviations, laboratory tests (data used when transcribing medical reports), and basic medical transcription guidelines.

Karonne J. Becklin
Edith M. Sunnarborg

CHAPTER 1

Introduction to Medical Transcription

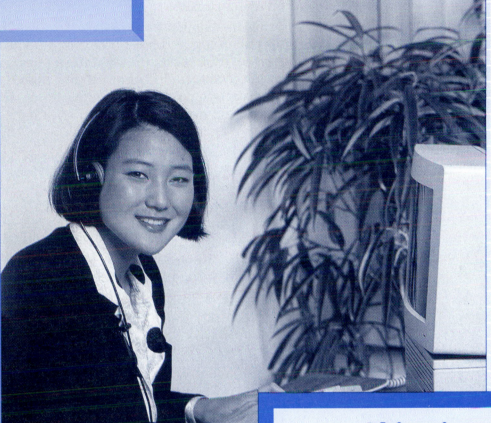

Medical transcriptionists are employed in a variety of settings. They may work for employers in hospitals, clinics, or physicians' offices. Opportunities are also available in firms that provide transcription services for hospitals and physicians. *In what setting do you think you would like to begin your career?*

Objectives

After completing this chapter, you will be able to

1. List four necessary skills of the entry-level medical transcriptionist.
2. List four personal attributes of a medical transcriptionist.
3. Describe the functions of AAMT.
4. Discuss the importance of professionalism.
5. List the process to become a certified medical transcriptionist.
6. Compare and contrast analog transcription and digital transcription.
7. Discuss how new technology will change the field of medical transcription.

A *medical transcriptionist* transcribes dictation by physicians and other health care professionals into comprehensive health care records. The term *medical language specialist* is also commonly used for this profession. The items that are transcribed are highly technical, containing medical terms. The dictation is also confidential. All medical documents must be prepared accurately, applying professional and ethical processes.

Medical transcriptionists must have practical knowledge of medical terminology, anatomy and physiology, disease processes, pharmaceutical terms, pathological and laboratory terms, and related medical terms. A successful transcriptionist also demonstrates correct English usage, applying proper grammar, punctuation, and style; proofing and editing; use of professional resources; listening skills; and word processing and computer functions as they relate to transcribing medical documents.

A medical transcriptionist who has a strong knowledge of a major word processing program can easily adapt to another word processing system or to a system that has been specifically developed for an individual medical facility. Also, medical transcriptionists must be highly motivated and self-disciplined, because they should be able to recognize discrepancies in dictation and appropriately edit and revise them or to obtain corrections from the appropriate person. For example, a transcribed chart note reads, "a 2.5-cm nodule in the right breast." The physician has also dictated a letter indicating that this patient has a nodule in the left breast. To resolve this discrepancy, the medical transcriptionist attached the chart note to the letter with a note to the physician asking which is correct.

The medical transcriptionist may work in a variety of health care facilities, such as hospitals, clinics, physician offices, transcription services, insurance companies, home health care facilities, laboratories, government medical facilities, legal offices, research centers, and other medically related facilities. Figure 1.1 defines many of the medical specialties and subspecialties that a medical transcriptionist might encounter.

There are prominent physical and mental demands in this profession. The medical transcriptionist must be an independent person who can work directly with the computer and transcribing process (see Figure 1.2 on page 4). Transcriptionists must also make efficient use of time, material, and resources; use sound judgment about when to seek assistance; recognize the ethical and legal nature of the work; be accurate and take the initiative to meet quantity demands; and demonstrate thoroughness, paying attention to details in the transcription process. The transcriptionist must learn to balance the use of earphones and foot control with keyboarding skills.

Figure 1.1

MEDICAL SPECIALTIES AND SUBSPECIALTIES

Allergy: An allergist diagnoses and treats adverse reactions to foods, drugs, and other substances.

Anesthesiology: An anesthesiologist maintains pain relief and stable body functions of patients during surgical procedures.

Dentistry: A dentist is concerned with the care and treatment of teeth and gums especially prevention, diagnosis, and treatment of deformities, diseases, and traumatic injuries. Subspecialties include:

An **endodontist** specializes in root canal work.

A **forensic** dentist applies dental facts to legal issues.

An **oral surgeon** specializes in jaw surgery and extractions.

An **orthodontist** straightens teeth.

A **pedodontist** provides dental care for children.

A **periodontist** specializes in gum disease.

A **prosthodontist** specializes in dentures and artificial teeth.

Dermatology: The dermatologist diagnoses and treats diseases of the skin and related tissues.

Emergency Medicine: An emergency room physician provides immediate treatment of accidents or illnesses.

Family Practice: A family practice physician provides total health care for the family.

Gynecology: A gynecologist is concerned with the diseases of the female genital tract as well as female endocrinology and reproductive physiology.

Internal Medicine: An internist diagnoses a wide range of nonsurgical illnesses. Subspecialties include:

Cardiovascular Medicine: A cardiologist diagnoses and treats diseases of the heart, blood vessels, and lungs.

Endocrinology: An endocrinologist diagnoses and treats endocrine gland diseases.

Gastroenterology: A gastroenterologist diagnoses and treats diseases of the digestive tract and related organs.

Gerontology: The gerontologist treats the process and problems of aging.

Hematology: A hematologist diagnoses and treats diseases of the blood.

Immunology: An immunologist diagnoses and treats symptoms of immunity, diseases, induced sensitivity, and allergies.

Infectious Disease: A specialist in infectious disease diagnoses and treats all types of infectious diseases.

Nephrology: A nephrologist diagnoses and treats disorders of the kidneys and related functions.

Oncology: An oncologist diagnoses and treats cancer.

Pulmonary Disease: A pulmonologist diagnoses and treats lung disorders.

Rheumatology: A rheumatologist is concerned with the study, diagnosis, and treatment of rheumatic conditions.

Neurology: A neurologist diagnoses and treats disorders of the nervous system.

Obstetrics: An obstetrician provides care during pregnancy and childbirth.

Occupational Medicine: A specialist in occupational medicine works with companies to prevent and manage occupational and environmental injury, illness and disability, and to promote health and productivity of workers and their families and communities.

Ophthalmology: An ophthalmologist cares for the eyes and the vision.

continued

MEDICAL SPECIALTIES AND SUBSPECIALTIES

Orthopedics: An orthopedic surgeon or orthopedist provides treatment of the musculoskeletal system.

Otorhinolaryngology: A physician in otorhinolaryngology specializes in the diagnosis and treatment of illnesses of the ears, nose, and throat (ENT).

Pathology: A pathologist investigates the causes of disease using laboratory techniques.

Pediatrics: A pediatrician specializes in the comprehensive treatment of children.

Physical Medicine/Rehabilitation: A physiatrist evaluates and treats all types of disease through physical means, such as heat.

Plastic Surgery: A plastic surgeon repairs and reconstructs body structures through surgical means.

Psychiatry: A psychiatrist diagnoses and treats mental, emotional, and behavioral disorders.

Radiology and Nuclear Medicine: A radiologist uses radioactive materials to diagnose and treat disease.

Thoracic Surgery: A thoracic surgeon uses surgery to diagnose or treat diseases of the chest.

Urology: A urologist diagnoses and treats diseases of the urinary tract.

Figure 1.2

A medical transcriptionist is usually equipped with a computer, earphones, and a foot pedal. *What is the purpose of each of these parts of the transcription system?*

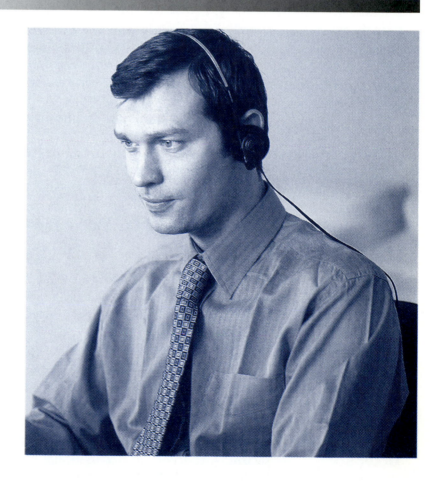

The working environment for medical transcription can vary greatly. Medical facilities have access to outside sources to recommend an ergonomic working environment. Ergonomic keyboards are available to ease hand and arm strain. A variety of desks, chairs, and lighting can ease the physical and mental demands of medical transcription.

1.2 American Association for Medical Transcription (AAMT)

The American Association for Medical Transcription (AAMT) represents the medical transcription profession, emphasizes continuing education, sponsors regular educational meetings and symposia, and promotes professionalism. The AAMT publishes a bimonthly magazine, *Journal of the American Association for Medical Transcription (JAAMT)*, with professional articles, advertisements, and information about AAMT activities. It is a worthwhile resource for students, instructors, and practicing transcriptionists.

Practicing medical transcriptionists need to make an effort to continue their education. The AAMT on the national, state, and local levels offers many opportunities for continuing education. The organization also offers educational products for educators.

American Association for Medical Transcription
100 Sycamore Avenue
Modesto, CA 95355-9690
Telephone: 209-551-0883
E-mail: aamt@aamt.org
Web: http://www.aamt.org

Job Descriptions

A model job description for medical transcriptionists created by the AAMT is shown in Appendix F. This description covers knowledge, skills, and abilities; working conditions; physical demands; and job responsibilities and performance standards. The AAMT Web site offers access to current information about the profession.

Code of Ethics

The AAMT Code of Ethics, shown in Figure 1.3 on page 6, evaluates the standards of conduct and professionalism for medical transcription.

Figure 1.3

AAMT CODE OF ETHICS

Part I   Association Membership

Preamble

Be aware that it is by our standards of conduct and professionalism that the American Association for Medical Transcription (AAMT) is evaluated. As members of AAMT we should recognize and observe the goals and objectives of the organization and the limitations and confinements imposed by its bylaws, policies and procedures.

Scope of Member Conduct

AAMT members (in individual categories of membership) will:

1. Place the goals and purposes of the Association above personal gain and work for the good of the profession.
2. Discharge honorably and to the best of their ability the responsibility of any elected or appointed Association position.
3. Preserve the confidential nature of professional judgments and determinations made confidentially by the official bodies of the Association.
4. Represent truthfully and accurately (a) one's membership in the Association, (b) one's roles and functions in the Association, and (c) any positions and decisions of the Association.

Part II   Professional Standards

Preamble

AAMT members are aware that it is by our standards of conduct and professionalism that the entire profession of medical transcription is evaluated. We should conduct ourselves in the practice of our profession so as to bring dignity and honor to ourselves and to the profession of medical transcription as medical language specialists. Therefore, the following standards are considered essential in the workplace:

1. A medical transcriptionist undertakes work only if she/he is competent to perform it.
2. A medical transcriptionist exhibits honesty and integrity in his/her professional work and activities.
3. A medical transcriptionist is reasonably familiar with and complies with principles of accuracy, authenticity, privacy, confidentiality, and security concerning patient care information.
4. A medical transcriptionist engages in professional reading and continuing education sufficient to stay abreast of important professional information.
5. A medical transcriptionist does not misrepresent or falsify information concerning medical records, his/her fees, work or professional experience, credentials, or affiliations.
6. A medical transcriptionist complies with applicable law and professional standards governing his/her work.
7. A medical transcriptionist does not assist others to violate ethical principles or professional standards of the medical transcription field.
8. If a medical transcriptionist learns of a significant unethical practice by another medical transcriptionist, she/he takes reasonable steps to resolve the matter.
9. A medical transcriptionist who agrees to serve in an official capacity in a professional association exhibits honesty and integrity in discharging his/her responsibilities.
10. AAMT members who are not medical transcriptionists should abide by the above principles where applicable.

Certification

The Medical Transcription Certification Commission (MTCC) is responsible for the credentialing program of the AAMT. Transcriptionists who want to attain the status of certified medical transcriptionist (CMT) voluntarily take a two-part examination. Part I consists of multiple-choice questions that assess essential knowledge and skills: medical terminology, English language and usage, anatomy and physiology, disease processes, health care record, and professional development. Part II contains a variety of medical reports and documents representing dictation from the medical specialties to be transcribed using appropriate references. The exam is available for a fee to any transcriptionist who feels ready to take it. Information is available on the AAMT Web site.

1.3 Transcription Process

Types of Dictation Systems

Medical transcriptionists may work with dictation that is stored on an audiocassette or a digitally stored recording. In a cassette system, the physician or health care professional dictates onto an audiocassette and physically transfers the audiocassette to the transcription area. This type of transcription is referred to as analog dictation. The medical transcriptionist works on a computer using a transcriber with earphones and a foot control.

There are many new, innovative programs for electronically enabled transcription. The physician may dictate to a digital dictation system via telephone. This dictation can be transcribed by the physician's facility-based transcriptionist, or it may be transcribed at an outside transcription service (referred to as "outsourcing"). The transcriptionist's computer has a modem or other online connection, earphones, and a foot control connected to it. Sounds are clearer in digital dictation, making transcription easier.

Digital dictation can be transferred to the medical transcriptionist via a modem using the telephone line or via the Internet, which eliminates long-distance costs. Digital dictation can be transcribed live or re-recorded for later use. Since the medical transcriptionist does not need to receive an audiocassette, it is possible to work within the dictating facility or at a remote location, including the transcriptionist's home. Digital dictation has allowed transcription to become a competitive international industry.

Figure 1.4

Physicians dictate using a variety of devices, such as handheld recorders. *What methods are used to transmit the dictation to the medical transcriptionist?*

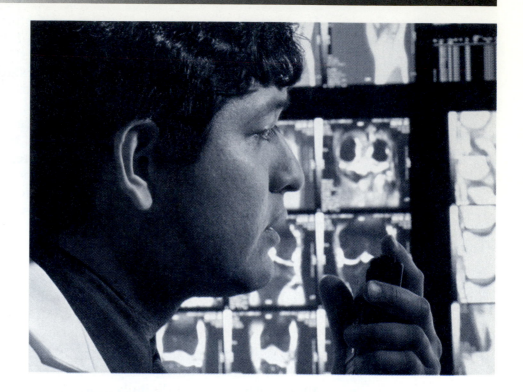

Speech Recognition

Speech recognition technology is also used in transcribing medical documents. A physician who has been trained in dictating can dictate into a software program that creates a document which can be printed or displayed on a computer screen. Speech recognition technology is not perfect, and the document is likely to contain errors. The medical transcriptionist edits and proofs the document, makes corrections, and produces the final copy. Medical transcription editors and proofers may work in offices, hospitals, or offsite locations.

Some speech recognition systems provide "fill-in-the-blank" technology that allows the user to touch the screen to select the necessary terms. These systems are used in places such as emergency rooms and for documenting obstetric, surgical, and routine physical examination procedures where repetitive questions have limited answer choices. For example, an emergency room physician may perform a quick assessment of unrelated systems for a patient with a urinary tract infection. The physician might select these systems, such as the cardiovascular system, on the computer screen, and then select the result of the examination, such as "findings negative."

There are software programs available to increase productivity, such as medical spelling checkers and expander software. Medical dictionaries can be purchased in CD-ROM format and loaded in the transcriber's computer. Also, as a transcriber confirms the spelling of a new term or drug, it can be added to the spelling checker.

Commercial medical expander programs allow dictation to be transcribed in a shorthand form such as keying *tp* for *the patient* or *wd* for *well developed*. The brief forms are transcribed into regular words with appropriate spacing and punctuation. These programs require the user to memorize many abbreviations, but they are generally user friendly with screen prompts. They can also be customized with the user's abbreviations. A home-based medical transcriptionist may have to purchase some of the software programs to aid in the transcription process.

1.4 Transcription Guidelines

Appendix A contains basic medical transcription guidelines to use in transcribing medical documents. These guidelines generally correlate with *The AAMT Book of Style for Medical Transcription*, which may be purchased from AAMT. The guidelines review punctuation, capitalization, abbreviations, numbers, and symbol usage as they apply to the transcription process. Medical transcriptionists at all levels should consult references as needed.

Figure 1.5

Many medical transcriptionists work for transcription service companies that employ workers who come in to the office or work at home. *What are the advantages and disadvantages of each of these work environments?*

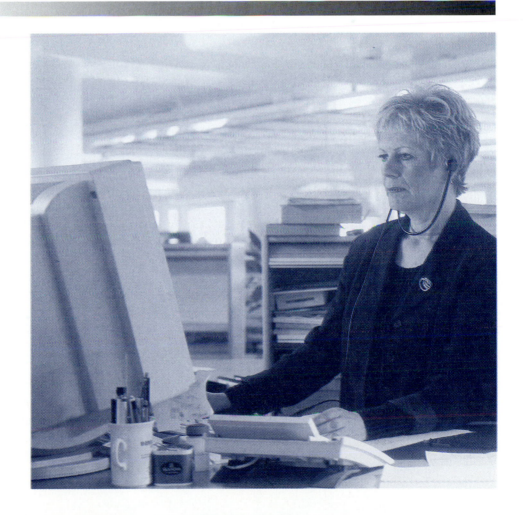

1.5 Quality Assurance

Effective quality assurance guidelines must be practiced in medical transcription. Generally, each facility sets quantity policies that are easily measured, evaluated, and controlled. There must also be a workable balance between quantity and quality requirements. Quality in medical transcription is usually measured by the correctness and appropriateness of the transcribed medical document. For example, it is critical to be accurate in the transcription of medication amounts.

The medical transcriptionist must have access to current references; adequate transcribing and computer equipment; a conducive work environment; efficient guidelines and procedures for transcribing, proofing, editing, and protecting confidentiality; and sufficient supervision.

Name _____ Date _____

Exercise 1.1 Building Your Knowledge of Medical Transcription

Directions Circle the correct answer for each of the following statements with a *T* for a true statement and an *F* for a false statement.

1. *Medical language specialist* is synonymous with *medical assistant.*　　　　　　　　　　　　　　　　T　　　F

2. A person must be trained in medical transcription before transcribing medical documents.　　　　　　　T　　　F

3. AAMT means American Association for Medical Transcription.　　　　　　　　　　　　　　　T　　　F

4. Medical documents that have been transcribed by a speech recognition system do not need to be proofed or edited.　　T　　　F

5. The main function of AAMT is to accredit medical transcription programs.　　　　　　　　　T　　　F

6. The certification exam for medical transcriptionists has two parts.　　　T　　　F

7. Digital dictation does not use an audiocassette.　　　T　　　F

8. Words cannot be added to medical speller software.　　　T　　　F

9. Medical expander software allows the user to input brief forms, which are transcribed into regular words.　　　T　　　F

10. Quantity of medical transcription is more important than quality standards.　　　T　　　F

Exercise 1.2 Researching Careers

Directions Using the Internet or newspapers, research medical transcription positions in your geographic location. State the job requirements and salary (if given), and describe the position.

Exercise 1.3 Using the Internet: Researching the AAMT

Directions Using the Internet (http://www.aamt.org), obtain the cost of student membership in the AAMT in your state. Using the same Web site, research Part I of the certification exam, listing the different areas covered and their corresponding percentages.

CHAPTER

2

The Patient's Medical Record

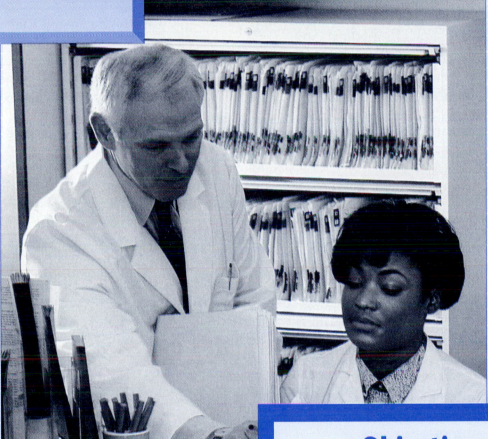

A person beginning the study of medical transcription may be overwhelmed by the strange spelling and pronunciation of medical terms. Approximately 75% of these terms are either Latin or Greek. New terms are constantly being formed as technologies advance. In a basic medical terminology course, you will have learned the foundation for medical word building. This knowledge will be used in transcribing patients' medical records. *What types of documents are typically part of a medical record?*

Objectives

After completing this chapter, you will be able to

1. State the essential components of a clinical data entry in the patient's record.
2. Identify abbreviations as they apply to the components of a physical examination.
3. List five types of records that may be found in the patient's chart.
4. Define the four methods of examination.
5. Explain the SOAP method of dictation.

2.1 Word Building

Medical record documentation is required to record the pertinent facts about the patient's health history. A medical transcriptionist must have a good understanding of medical language to ensure the accuracy of the medical record.

Prefixes and Suffixes

These word elements—prefixes and suffixes—are commonly found in medical data:

Prefixes		Prefixes		Prefixes	
a, an	without, lack of	endo	within	post	after, behind
ab	away from	epi	on, upon	pre	before
ad	toward	ex	outside	retro	behind
ante	before	hemi	half	semi	half
anti	against	hyper	above, excessive	sub	under
bi	twice, double	hypo	under, deficient	super/supra	upper, excessive
contra	against	inter	between	trans	across
dys	abnormal, pain	intra	within		

Diagnostic Suffixes		Operative Suffixes		Symptomatic Suffixes	
-cele	herniation	-centesis	puncture	-algia	pain
-emia	blood condition	-ectomy	remove	-lysis	break up, dissolve
-iasis	condition	-plasty	formation		
-itis	inflammation	-rrhagia	hemorrhage		
-megaly	enlargement	-rrhaphy	suture		
-oma	tumor	-scopy	examine		
-opia	vision	-stomy	new opening		
-osis	abnormal condition	-tomy	cut into		
-pathy	disease	-tripsy	crush		
-trophy	nourish				

Directional Terms

The following directional terms are frequently used in patient documentation:

TERM	MEANING
anterior/ventral	toward the front
posterior/dorsal	toward the back
horizontal/transverse	across
vertical	up and down
inferior	below
superior	above
medial	middle
lateral	side
proximal	nearer to point of origin
distal	away from point of origin
symmetric	equal

Types of Movement

Another common set of terms involves types of movement. The following items, illustrated in Figure 2.1 on page 16, are often found in patient medical records.

TERM	MEANING
abduction	moves away from the body
adduction	moves toward the midline of the body
circumduction (of the shoulders and hips)	allows movement in a circle
extension	increases the size of an angle
flexion	decreases the size of an angle
eversion	turns outward
inversion	turns inward
pronation (of the forearm)	places the palm down
supination (of the forearm)	places the palm up
recumbent	lying down, reclining
rotation	moves the head from side to side

Figure 2.1

Common Movement
of the Joints

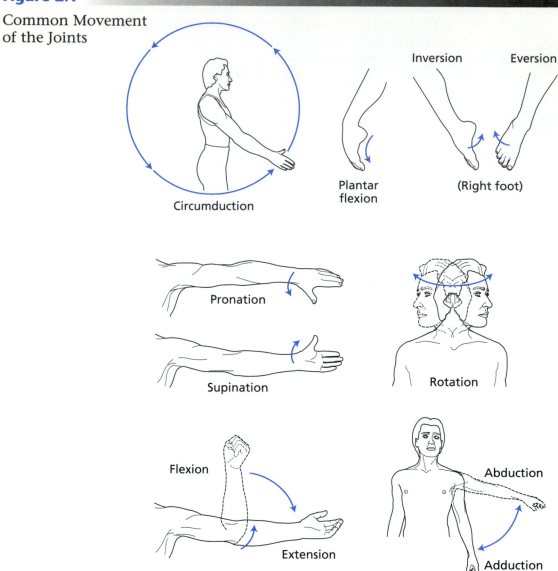

Circumduction

Plantar
flexion

Inversion   Eversion

(Right foot)

Pronation

Supination

Rotation

Flexion

Extension

Abduction

Adduction

2.2   Clinical Data

Clinical data are information about a patient's condition. They are
entered or noted each time the patient visits the office or is seen
by the physician in another location, such as a hospital or nursing
home. Entries include the date of the visit, data pertaining to
the visit, and the name of the person who saw or examined
the patient.

The physician may use any of a variety of systems to record the
medical data of patients. The patient's *medical record*—also called
the *chart* or *file*—is an accumulation of all data pertaining to that
patient. The patient medical record (PMR) may include any of the
following documents:

History and physical examination

Chart notes made by the physician, nurse, or other health care provider

Laboratory and x-ray reports

Special procedure reports

Correspondence

Forms used for a specific purpose, such as immunization records, developmental and growth records of children, preemployment physicals, preoperative physicals, disability reports, and burn or injury diagrams

2.3   Methods of Examination

The reason for the patient's encounter with the physician—whether a routine checkup or a complaint—is evaluated by the provider. Different methods are used, depending on the nature of the encounter. Four principal means of examining a patient are as follows:

- **Observation/inspection** The examiner observes the general appearance including hygiene and grooming, general state of health, posture, mannerisms, and obvious deformities of the patient.

- **Percussion** Tapping (*percussion*) with the fingers or small hammer produces sounds that help to determine size, position, or density of an underlying organ (*viscera*).

- **Palpation** *Palpation* refers to the sense of touch and may be used to determine the condition of an underlying organ.

- **Auscultation** By listening to sounds, usually with a stethoscope, the examiner may determine sounds in the heart, lungs, or abdomen.

2.4   Documentation

Because it is the legal record of the care the physician provides and may need to be reviewed by others in the course of the patient's treatment, the medical record should be complete and legible. The documentation of each patient encounter (visit) should include the chief complaint and/or reason for the visit, physical findings, diagnostic test results, clinical impression or diagnosis, and plan for care.

Each notation begins with a statement about why the patient is seeking the physician's advice. This reason for the visit may be stated as a symptom or sign and may be referred to as the *chief complaint (CC), problem,* or *subjective.*

A complete physical examination is very detailed and generally follows a specific format, such as this:

History of present illness (HPI) or *subjective* is information given by the patient. This information includes a description of symptoms and when they began, associated factors, and remedies tried.

Past medical history (PMH) includes illness, injuries, and surgeries the patient may have had as well as any allergies to medications or to other substances.

Family history (FH) consists of information about the health of the patient's blood relatives that might be significant to the patient's condition.

Social history (SH) and *marital history* are included if pertinent to the patient's treatment. The social history may include eating, drinking, and smoking habits, as well as occupation and interests of the patient.

(*Note:* PMI, FH, and SH are sometimes abbreviated as *PFSH* and combined into one entry.)

Review of systems (ROS) includes a review in which the physician asks specific questions about the functioning of each body system.

Objective or *physical examination (PE)* provides an examination record. Laboratory and x-ray findings are also considered objective information, although they are usually placed in a separate paragraph.

Diagnosis, assessment, impression, appraisal, or *conclusion* provides the examining physician's interpretation of the information. Further study may be needed, in which case the diagnosis may be *rule out (R/O), suspected,* or *probable,* and additional studies will be planned.

Plan, disposition, treatment, recommendations, or *advice* include instructions to the patient, additional investigation procedures to be performed, medications prescribed, and so forth.

Heading Sequence

Figure 2.2 on page 20 shows an example of documentation of a patient's visit. The seqence of headings for a complete history and physical examination may be as follows:

CHIEF COMPLAINT

HISTORY OF PRESENT ILLNESS

PAST MEDICAL HISTORY

ALLERGIES

MEDICATIONS

SURGERIES

FAMILY HISTORY

SOCIAL HISTORY

REVIEW OF SYSTEMS

PHYSICAL EXAMINATION

GENERAL
HEENT
NECK
CHEST
LUNGS
HEART
ABDOMEN
PELVIC
RECTAL
EXTREMITIES
NEUROLOGIC

IMPRESSION

PLAN

Figure 2.2

HISTORY AND PHYSICAL

Joseph Iverson   4/22/20—

CHIEF COMPLAINT: Joe is a new patient who presents to the clinic with left knee pain, swelling, and weakness. He denies previous trauma to this area but has had right knee pain and arthritis in past. Recently he changed physicians because of change in health care policies.

PAST MEDICAL HISTORY: Negative.

ALLERGIES: None.

MEDICATIONS: None.

PAST SURGICAL HISTORY: Negative.

SOCIAL HISTORY: Nonsmoker. He does drink beer, 4 to 6 cans per day.

FAMILY HISTORY: Father has degenerative disk disease; brother had herniated disk which required a laminectomy.

EXAM:
Weight 304 pounds. Initial BP 134/104; repeat 132/94.
SKIN: Flushed and red.
LEFT KNEE: Exam showed the knee to be warm and swollen compared to right knee. Extension is 180 degrees; flexion is 90 degrees. Negative drawer, Apley grind, and patellar apprehension test. He has marked tenderness and crepitus in the patellar and supra-patellar ligaments on palpation.
PERIPHERAL PULSES: They are 2+/4 and symmetrical in the popliteal, posterior tibial, and dorsalis pedis areas.

X-RAY: No gross evidence of fractures or abnormalities.

LAB: Nonfasting glucose 120, total cholesterol 253, and uric acid 8.8.

DIAGNOSIS: Left knee pain and swelling secondary to gouty arthritis.

PLAN: Daypro 600 mg 2 daily for 1 week. Decrease alcohol consumption. Recheck in 1 week; if there is no improvement, he will start on allopurinol.

John Blackburn, MD/xx

2.5 | Narrative Notes

An examination for a routine office visit other than a physical exam is limited to the immediate complaint or symptom. Routine office visits may also be referred to as checkups, rechecks, or progress notes. For example, the note may read that a patient returned for a recheck of ears or for a blood pressure check.

Each facility has its own format for transcribing physicians' dictation. One of the most common formats is the SOAP method, which has four essential components.

1. *Subjective (S)* findings—what the patient tells the examiner about the problem or complaint.

2. *Objective (O)* findings—what the examiner discovers on examination; may include laboratory, x-ray, or other diagnostic procedures.

3. *Assessment (A)*—the diagnosis or diagnoses based on the above findings.

4. *Plan (P)*—a course of treatment, such as further laboratory or x-ray studies, surgery, medications, referral, and so forth.

The facility may have a preference for using either complete headings or abbreviations with the SOAP format (see Figure 2.3).

Figure 2.3

CHART NOTE

Raymond Piper   4/26/20—

SUBJECTIVE
The mother brought in this 1-month-old male. The patient is doing very well. They have been using the phototherapy blanket. He is thirsty, has good yellow stooling, and continues on formula. His alertness is normal. Other pertinent ROS is noncontributory.

OBJECTIVE
Afebrile. Comfortable. Jaundice is only minimal at this time. No scleral icterus. Good activity level. Normal fontanel. TMs, nose, mouth, pharynx, neck, heart, lungs, abdomen, liver, spleen, and groins are normal. Normal cord care and circumcision. Good extremities.

ASSESSMENT
Resolving physiologic jaundice on phototherapy.

PLAN
Will stop phototherapy and do a bilirubin level in a couple of days to make sure there is no rebound. The patient is to be seen in one week. Push fluids. Routine care was discussed.

Debra Litman, MD/xx

Each entry in a chart should end with a signature line. This sign-off varies according to the policy of the clinic or doctor. The physician's or dictator's name may be followed by the initials of the transcriptionist. The signature should start at the left margin, and three blank lines should be left for the actual signature. The signature line may also include the date of dictation (D) and transcription (T).

Debra Litman, MD/kb

Lee W. Kim, MD/kb   D: 10/20/20—   T: 10/21/20—

2.6 Your Transcribing Instructions

The medical reports in this text-workbook represent dictation that is given in physicians' offices and clinics. The types of reports include chart notes, progress notes, history and physical reports, x-ray reports, procedure notes, and consultations.

Formats

In an office or clinic, transcription is often keyed directly onto sheets of paper, continuing from visit to visit with about one-half inch of space between reports. Another method is to use shingles, which are individual paper forms that are keyed onto and then inserted separately into the patient's chart. In this text, you will key each document on a separate sheet, as directed by your instructor.

Document formats vary from office to office. For this text, unless otherwise directed by your instructor, follow the models shown in Figures 2.4 (on page 23), 2.5 (on page 24), 2.6 (on page 25), and 2.7 (on page 26) plus the history and physical model shown in Figure 2.2 on page 20 and the SOAP model in Figure 2.3 on page 21. These models are generally similar to the AAMT's preferred styles.

Figure 2.4

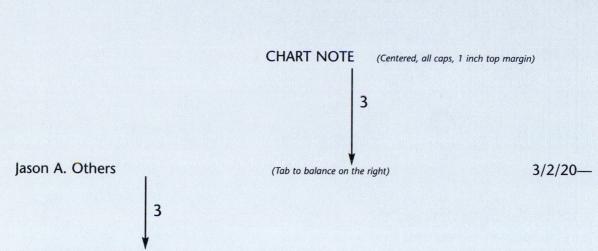

CHART NOTE   *(Centered, all caps, 1 inch top margin)*

3

Jason A. Others   *(Tab to balance on the right)*   3/2/20—

3

HISTORY OF PRESENT ILLNESS
This patient developed some burning sensation when urinating, followed by pain and hematuria. There was no penile discharge.

PHYSICAL EXAMINATION
BP 189/70. Pulse 95. Temperature 96.5°F.

ABDOMEN: Soft with slight discomfort to palpation in the hypogastric region. No CVA tenderness.

SCROTUM AND PENIS: Appear normal without discharge.

LAB
Urinalysis shows brown color, cloudy, and ketones small. Specific gravity 1.021. WBC 50-75, RBC packed, and moderate bacteria. Culture was sent to outside lab.

DIAGNOSIS
Cystitis.

TREATMENT
The patient is ALLERGIC TO SULFA. Therefore, Amoxicillin 250 mg t.i.d. x 10 days and Pyridium one tablet t.i.d. #6 were prescribed. The patient is to force fluids to 2000 cc daily and is to call for culture results in 2 days. Scheduled followup in 10 days.

3

Lee W. Kim, MD/xx *(Transcriptionist's initials)*

Figure 2.5

WILCOX MEDICAL CENTER
6210 Eagle Street
Denver, CO 80239-7145

303-555-1026   Fax: 303-555-9320

March 21, 20—   *(Start on line two inches)*

National Handicap Housing, Inc.
1050 South Fillmore Street
Denver, CO 80209-6578

Ladies and Gentlemen

RE: Keith Atwood   Patient #123-403

Mr. Atwood has been struggling with physical difficulties as well as with depression. During the time that I have seen him, he has been diligent in following up with appointments. His best period of sustained function occurred when he had a stable home life. During the past several months, he has had to make several residential moves. It is my opinion that this has exacerbated his condition both from physical and mental standpoints.

I would support any efforts to find permanent housing for him. Given his inability to work over the past several years, I believe that he would be a good candidate for low-income housing.

Please contact me if you have any additional concerns about Mr. Atwood's condition.

Sincerely

John Blackburn, MD

xx

LETTER EXAMPLE: Full block format, open punctuation. (*Note:* The standard punctuation style has a colon after the salutation and a comma after the complimentary closing.)

Headings

Some guidelines call for section headings followed by colons and information continuing on the same line, thus saving space on the medical document.

PAST MEDICAL HISTORY: Negative.

FAMILY HISTORY: Father has degenerative disk disease; brother had herniated disk that required a laminectomy.

Your Work Setting

In this text-workbook, you are employed as a transcriptionist by the Wilcox Medical Center, 6210 Eagle Street, Denver, Colorado 80239-7145. The physicians are John Blackburn, MD, family practice; Lee W. Kim, MD, internal medicine; Debra Litman, MD, family practice; and Lynn Solinski, MD, internal medicine. The complete headings are used for the SOAP format. Use this style in preparing each type of report.

Figure 2.6

X-RAY REPORT

Kate Gonsinski   12/3/20—

BILATERAL MAMMOGRAM
There is irregularly dense glandular tissue throughout both breasts. There are no suspicious masses or calcifications seen. There is no radiographic evidence of malignancy. There has been no significant change compared with the previous study dated May 19, 20—.

CONCLUSION
Negative mammogram.

Karen Twan, MD/xx

Figure 2.7

PROCEDURE NOTE

Pamela W. Evanston   12/19/20—

PROCEDURE
Colposcopy.

INDICATIONS FOR PROCEDURE
In October of this year, patient had a low-grade epithelial lesion of undetermined significance, probably mild dysplasia or CIN grade 1 with HPV effect. For that reason, we scheduled her for colposcopy.

Patient is 21 years old, para 1-0-0-1. Her age at first pregnancy was 19. She has no history of venereal disease or sexually transmitted infection.

PROCEDURE
After discussion of procedure, risks, benefits, and possible alternatives, patient gave written consent for the procedure.

Speculum was placed in the vagina and cervix brought into view. After applying vinegar, we saw a large transformation zone consisting of white epithelium with mosaic at 12 and 1 o'clock and punctation and mosaic at 5–6 o'clock. It was more extensive on the posterior cervix, but it went circumferentially and under the anterior cervix, possibly inside the os. Endocervical biopsies were done at 12 and 1 and at 5 and 6 o'clock. They were sent separately to pathology.

DIAGNOSIS
Colposcopy for abnormal Pap smear.

PLAN
We will await pathology results of biopsies. Then we will recommend either cryocautery or loop electrosurgical excision procedure based on the severity of findings.

Les Perez, MD/xx

2.7 General Terms

KEY_terms_ The following general terms may be found throughout transcription. Practice word recognition and pronunciation; then spell each term. The macron (ˉ) is used for long vowels, and the breve (˘) is used for short vowels and for the indefinite vowel sound of the schwa (∂). Stressed syllables are followed by a prime (´). A hyphen separates the syllables. A review of medication abbreviations is placed throughout the transcription.

TERM	PRONUNCIATION	MEANING
ache	(āk)	pain that persists
acute	(ă-kyūt´)	having a short and sharp course
adolescent	(ad-ō-les´ent)	person in the teen years
afebrile	(ā-feb´ril)	not having an elevated body temperature
allergy	(al´er-jē)	sensitivity to a substance that results in symptoms
ambulate	(am´byū-lāt)	to walk about
anomaly	(ă-nom´ă´-lē)	abnormality; deviation from normal
asepsis	(ă-sep´sis)	cleanliness
atrophy	(at´rō-fē)	wasting of a structure
benign	(bē-nīn´)	of mild character
breadth	(bretth)	width
calcification	(kal´si-fi-kā´shŭn)	deposit of lime or calcium salt
catheter	(kath´ĕ-ter)	tubular instrument to allow passage of air or fluid
chronic	(kron´ik)	marked by slow progress and long continuance
congenital	(kon-jen´i-tăl)	existing at birth
constriction	(kon-strik´shŭn)	tightening, squeezing, contracting, or narrowing
contaminate	(kon-tam´i-nāt)	to render unclean
contraindication	(kon-tră-in-di-kā´shŭn)	inadvisable
crisis	(krī´sis)	a sudden change
curettage	(kyū-rĕ-tahzh´)	scraping of the interior of a cavity
debris	(dĕ-brē´)	material that does not belong in that area
dehydration	(dē-hī-drā´shŭn)	reduction of water content
diaphoresis	(dī´ă-fō-rē´sis)	perspiration; sweating
dilate	(dī´lāt)	to widen
disease	(di-zēz´)	illness
disposition	(dis-pŏ-zish´ŭn)	treatment or management
distention	(dis-ten´shŭn)	the state of being stretched or distended
elicit	(ĭ-lis´it)	reveal; provide
etiology	(ē´tē-ol´ō-jē)	study of cause of disease
hypertrophy	(hī-per´trō-fē)	increase in size of an organ
immobile	(im-mō´bil)	not capable of moving

TERM	PRONUNCIATION	MEANING
infection	(in-fek´shŭn)	invasion of area with pathogenic microorganisms
inflammation	(in-flă-mā´shŭn)	tissue reaction to injury (pain, warmth, swelling, redness)
injury	(in´jer-ē)	damage; trauma
malignant	(mă-lig´nănt)	harmful; causing death
manual	(man´yŭ-wăl)	pertaining to the hand
metastasis	(mĕ-tas´tă-sis)	spread of disease to another body part
nausea	(naw´zē-ă)	feeling of having to vomit
necrosis	(nĕ-krō´sis)	dead tissue; not viable
obese	(ō-bēs´)	excessively fat
obstruction	(ob-strŭk´shŭn)	blockage
occlusion	(ŏ-klū´shŭn)	closed
paroxysm	(par´ok-sizm)	spasm; sudden recurrence
postural	(pos´tyū-răl)	pertaining to position or posture
prognosis	(prog-nō´sis)	the outcome
prophylaxis	(prō-fi-lak´sis)	prevention
prosthesis	(pros´thē-sis)	artificial substitute for missing part
provisional	(prŏ-vi´zhŭ-năl)	temporary
purulent	(pyūr´ŭ-lent)	containing pus
quadrant	(kwah´drant)	quarter of a section
radiate	(rā´dē-āt)	to spread
recur	(rē-kŭr´)	to happen again
regimen	(rej´i-men)	program or plan
retention	(rē-ten´shŭn)	keeping in
sensitivity	(sen-si-tiv´i-tē)	responding to
septic	(sep´tik)	not clean; contaminated
sibling	(sib´ling)	offspring of the same parents
specimen	(spes´ĭ-men)	sample
stat	(stat)	right now
stenosis	(ste-nō´sis)	narrowing
sterile	(ster´il)	free of all microorganisms and spores
stricture	(strik´chŭr)	narrowing of hollow structure
suture	(sū´chŭr)	noun: threadlike material, stitch; verb: to sew or stitch
symptom	(simp´tŏm)	sign
syndrome	(sin´drōm)	group of signs or symptoms
therapy	(ther´ă-pē)	treatment
tract	(trakt)	pathway
trauma	(traw´mă)	injury

2.8 Build Your Editing Skills

In this section, you will gain the skills you need to correctly transcribe medical documents.

Selecting the Right Word

The words listed here are often confused in transcription because they sound alike when dictated but have different meanings. Study the words carefully so you will be able to select the correct term according to the context of the dictation.

TERM	MEANING	EXAMPLE
affect	make an impression	The patient was affected by the change in doctors.
	cause a result	This medication will affect the patient's energy.
	cause a change	The disease affected the patient's mind.
effect	result produced	This lab test has no effect on the total cost.
	general appearance	The effect of the new treatment plan will be known soon.
	become operative	The new fees will go in effect next month.
access	to approach	The patient has access to his or her chart through the physician.
	to consult	Access the data bank to obtain that information.
assess	to evaluate	The doctor assessed the damage.
	to set value or impose a charge	The doctor was assessed a $500 charge for incomplete records.
excess	to be greater than	We have in excess of 300 outdated patient brochures.

Using the Correct Punctuation

Medical transcriptionists use correct punctuation when preparing medical documents. Review the following punctuation guidelines. (The basic medical transcription guidelines appear in Appendix A.)

GUIDELINE	EXAMPLE
Separate equal adjectives (modifiers) with commas.	This was a middle-aged, malnourished white female.
Express ages in figures when used as significant statistics.	This 18-year-old patient was admitted to the hospital.
Use Arabic numbers with technical measurements.	The doctor found a 5-cm lesion on the patient's left leg.

Name _____ Date _____

Exercise 2.1 Building Your Medical Vocabulary

Directions Match each term from Column 2 with the appropriate meaning in Column 1.

Column 1   **Column 2**

____ 1. No lymph gland enlargement was felt.   **a.** assessment/diagnosis

____ 2. Rest, fluid, Tylenol for comfort. *(chart note)*   **b.** auscultation

____ 3. Patient complains of breathing difficulty.   **c.** objective
         (chart note)

____ 4. Noted rash across trunk.   **d.** observation

____ 5. No heart murmur was heard.   **e.** palpation

____ 6. Lungs are clear with good air entry. *(chart note)* **f.** percussion

____ 7. Tapping of abdomen produces a dull sound.   **g.** plan/treatment

____ 8. Upper respiratory tract infection. *(chart note)*   **h.** subjective

Name _____ Date _____

Exercise 2.2 Working with Drug Classifications

Directions Match each medication classification listed in Column 2 with its application in Column 1. (Use Appendix C, Drug Classifications, if necessary.)

Column 1	Column 2
____ 1. used to treat allergic-type symptoms	a. analgesic
____ 2. loosens respiratory secretions	b. anesthetic
____ 3. prevents clotting of blood	c. antacid
____ 4. causes blood vessels to widen	d. antibiotic
____ 5. decreases blood cholesterol	e. anticoagulant
____ 6. causes loss of sensation	f. antidepressant
____ 7. opens air passageways	g. antidiarrheal
____ 8. used to treat diarrhea	h. antidote
____ 9. relieves pain	i. antihistamine
____ 10. causes vomiting	j. bronchodilator
____ 11. relieves stomach acid	k. decongestant
____ 12. used to treat bacterial infection	l. diuretic
____ 13. given to counteract poison	m. emetic
____ 14. mood elevator	n. expectorant
____ 15. increases urinary output	o. hypolipidemic
____ 16. assists in getting rid of phlegm	p. laxative
____ 17. used to treat constipation	q. sedative
____ 18. quiets a patient	r. stimulant
____ 19. increases activity	s. vasodilator

Exercise 2.3 Building Terminology

Directions Match each prefix or suffix from Column 2 with its definition in Column 1.

Column 1	Column 2
____ 1. abnormal or painful	a. -algia
____ 2. across (from one to another)	b. ante
____ 3. after	c. anti
____ 4. against (bacteria)	d. bi
____ 5. before	e. -cele
____ 6. blood condition	f. -centesis
____ 7. condition	g. dys
____ 8. development or nourishment	h. -ectomy
____ 9. disease	i. -emia
____ 10. dissolve; break up (material)	j. ex
____ 11. enlargement	k. hyper
____ 12. examine visually	l. hypo
____ 13. excision or removal	m. intra
____ 14. hemorrhage	n. -itis
____ 15. incision into	o. -lysis
____ 16. inflammation	p. -megaly
____ 17. larger than normal	q. -oma
____ 18. less than normal	r. -opia
____ 19. outside (forces)	s. -osis
____ 20. pain	t. -pathy
____ 21. permanent new opening	u. -plasty
____ 22. pertaining to vision	v. post
____ 23. protrusion	w. -rrhagia
____ 24. reconstruction	x. -rrhaphy
____ 25. surgical crushing	y. -scopy
____ 26. surgical puncture	z. -stomy
____ 27. suture	aa. -tomy
____ 28. tumor	bb. trans
____ 29. twice	cc. -tripsy
____ 30. within (muscle)	dd. -trophy

Exercise 2.4 Using Directional and Movement Terms

Directions Fill in the blanks by using the following directional and movement terms.

abduction	dorsal	inferior	rotation
adduction	ventral	superior	symmetric
anterior	lateral	inversion	
posterior	extension	eversion	
distal	flexion	recumbent	
medial	horizontal	prone	
proximal	vertical	supine	

There is pain on (**1**)_____ (straightening) of the arm; (**2**)_____ (bending) is to 90°.

(**3**)_____ (moving head side to side) is limited by pain.

The breasts are (**4**)_____ (equal on both sides).

Patient was placed in the (**5**)_____ (flat on back) position, then rolled to the

(**6**)_____ (on the tummy) position after induction of anesthesia. He will

remain in the (**7**)_____ (lying down) position for 24 hours postoperatively.

There is pain in the (**8**)_____ (front) but not in the (**9**)_____ (back) lower rib region.

(**10**)_____ (raising the arm out from the body) causes shoulder pain;

(**11**)_____ (bringing arm toward the body) is negative.

The laceration extends from the (**12**)_____ (attachment to hand) through

the (**13**)_____ (middle) and into the (**14**)_____ (tip) of the finger.

Patient has tenderness along the (**15**)_____ (side) aspect of the palm; it does

not extend into the (**16**)_____ (back) aspect of the hand or into the

(**17**)_____ (palmar) aspect.

Pain is elicited with (**18**)_____ (pointing toes outward), but not with

(**19**)_____ (pointing toes inward).

Many blood vessels have (**20**)_____ (lower) segments and (**21**)_____ (anatomically higher or above) segments.

Sutures may be placed in a (**22**)_____ (crosswise) orientation or in a

(**23**)_____ (lengthwise to the body) one.

Exercise 2.5 Working with Abbreviations

Directions Using Appendix B, Abbreviations, define the following abbreviations.

TERM	DEFINITION
1. cm	_____
2. mm	_____
3. mcg	_____
4. mg	_____
5. g or gm	_____
6. kg	_____
7. mL	_____
8. cc	_____
9. q.d.	_____
10. q.o.d.	_____
11. q.h.	_____
12. q.2h.	_____
13. b.i.d.	_____
14. q.i.d.	_____
15. t.i.d.	_____
16. stat	_____
17. p.r.n.	_____
18. IM	_____
19. IV	_____
20. subq or subcu	_____
21. p.o.	_____
22. n.p.o.	_____

Exercise 2.6 Applying Your Editing Skill

Directions Circle the correct answer in each of the following sentences.

1. The physician's assistant has *access / assess / excess* to the patient's chart.

2. If the doctor operates, how will this *affect / effect* the patient's job?

3. The patient was found to be driving in *access / assess / excess* of 60 mph before the accident.

4. The doctor will *access / assess / excess* the patient's condition before discharging the patient to the nursing facility.

5. We will not know the *affect / effect* of the operation for 2 or 3 weeks.

6. The *38 year old / 38-year-old* patient was denied insurance coverage.

7. This *well-developed, / well-developed* Caucasian male was seen for acute chest pain.

8. The surgeon inserted a *three-cm / 3-cm* drain.

9. The physician gave us a *long, interesting / long interesting* lecture.

10. This is a *20-month-old, well-nourished / 20-month-old, well-nourished,* Caucasian male.

HINTS FOR TRANSCRIPTION

Before you begin the transcription for this chapter, be sure you know the following items:

- The format for a history and physical examination
- The format for a chart note
- Letter format
- The abbreviations shown in Appendix B

MEDICAL DOCUMENT TRANSCRIPTION

You are now ready to transcribe the dictation for Chapter 2.

The dictation for this chapter is by John Blackburn, MD. Use styles shown in this chapter with 1-inch left and right margins. Check with your instructor regarding whether you may key several reports on the same sheet of paper. Each report should include chapter and item number in the upper right corner as well as your name and the current date.

Chapter 2, Item 1
Your Name
Current Date

---

2 TRANSCRIPTION CHECKOFF SHEET

Use the transcription checkoff sheet to record your work and track your progress as a medical transcriptionist.

DOCTOR DICTATING John Blackburn, MD

TYPE OF DICTATION Chart notes, x-ray report, history and physical, and letters

DATE OF TRANSCRIPTION April 2, 20—

Item Number	Patient	Date Started	Date Completed	Grade/ Number of Errors
2.1	Carl Adams			
2.2	Cecelia Wert			
2.3	David Mendez			
2.4	David Mendez			
2.5	Letter to Ms. Mabel Ryerson, 13949 Adams Circle, Denver, CO 80241-3820			
2.6	Alison Beckman			
2.7	Michael Weysik			
2.8	Reis Olsson			
2.9	Letter to Susan Yee Yang			
2.10	Letter to Mr. Andrew Frank, ABC Construction Company, 750 South Fillmore Street, Denver, CO 80209-5072 RE: Warren Thomas			

CHAPTER 3

The Integumentary System

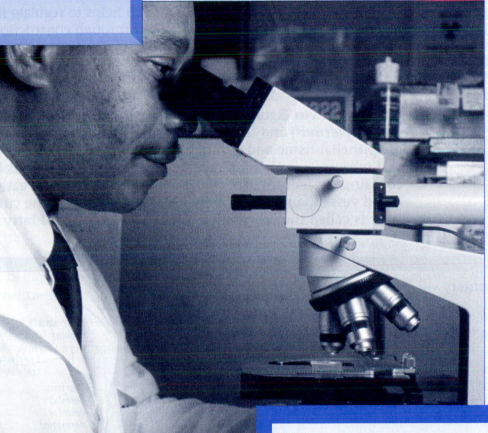

The skin holds the body together. It is the first line of defense against disease. Skin cancer is the most common cancer of men. The incidence of skin cancer has increased dramatically over the past several decades, primarily because of cumulative exposure to ultraviolet rays of the sun. Biopsies are examined by pathologists for indications of disease. *What other methods are used to gather information about patients' integumentary systems?*

Objectives

After completing this chapter, you will be able to

1. Use correct terms when transcribing medical documents covering integumentary system functions, assessment, conditions, procedures, and medications.
2. Match symptoms with the correct conditions.
3. Apply appropriate AAMT style guidelines to edit and format medical documents.

3.3 Symptoms and Disease Conditions

KEY *terms* The following symptoms and disease conditions apply to the integumentary system. Each term on this list is pronounced at the beginning of the dictation for this chapter. Study the list carefully, practicing pronunciation and building word recognition. Be sure you can spell each term correctly.

TERM	PRONUNCIATION	DEFINITION
abrasion	(ă-brā´zhun)	removal of superficial layer of skin
abscess	(ab´ses)	localized collection of pus
acne	(ak´nē)	inflammation of sebaceous glands
basal cell carcinoma	(bā´săl) (kar-si-nō´mă)	skin cancer
blister	(blis´ter)	fluid-filled structure under the skin
boil	(boyl)	infection in a hair follicle
cellulitis	(sel-yū-lī´tis)	inflammation of skin and subcutaneous tissue
comedos	(kom´ē-dōz)	blackheads caused by plugged oil gland
contusion	(kon-tū´shŭn)	bruise
cyst	(sist)	sac containing fluid
dermatitis	(der-mă-tī´tis)	general term indicating inflammation of skin
ecchymosis	(ek-i-mō´sis)	black and blue or purple discoloration of skin caused by bruise
eruption	(ē-rŭp´shŭn)	rash
erythema	(er-i-thē´mă)	reddish color to skin
excoriation	(eks-kō´rē-ā´shŭn)	break in skin caused by surface trauma; scratch
fissure	(fish´ŭr)	furrow; crack
fluctuant	(flŭk´tyū-ănt)	wavelike motion
herpes	(her´pēz)	eruption of vesicles on reddish bases caused by a virus
impetigo	(im-pe-tī´gō)	contagious superficial infection with vesicles and yellowish crusting
indurated	(in´dū-rāt-ed)	hardened or firm
keloid	(kē´loyd)	overgrowth of scar tissue
laceration	(las-er-ā´shŭn)	accidental tear of skin
lesion	(lē´zhŭn)	injury or pathological change in tissue

TERM	PRONUNCIATION	DEFINITION
maculae	(mak´yū-lē)	colored spots on skin
nevus	(nē´vŭs)	circumscribed, pigmented (shade of brown) area of skin; mole
nodule	(nod´yūl)	knob, mass, or swelling
papule	(pap´yūl)	pimple
paronychia	(par-ō-nik´ē-ă)	inflammation of the nail fold
pediculosis	(pě-dik´yū-lō´sis)	lice
plantar wart	(plan´tăr)	wart on sole of foot
pruritus	(prū-rī´tŭs)	itching
purulent	(pyūr´ŭ-lent)	containing pus
pustule	(pŭs´chŭl)	pimple with pus
scabies	(skā´bēz)	eruption caused by mite, which lays eggs in burrows under skin, with intense itching
seborrhea	(seb-ō-rē´ă)	overproduction of sebum from sebaceous glands, producing oily skin
verruca	(vě-rū´kă)	overgrowth of dermis, caused by virus; wart
vesicle	(ves´i-kl)	circumscribed elevation of skin containing fluid

3.4 Medical and Surgical Procedures

KEYterms The procedural terms that appear in the dictation for this chapter are described below. Study each term's spelling, pronunciation, and meaning so that you are prepared for transcription.

TERM	PRONUNCIATION	MEANING
biopsy	(bī´op-sē)	removing tissue for examination
cautery	(kaw´ter-ē)	agent (heat, cold, electric current, or chemical) used to burn tissue
cryosurgery	(krī-ō-ser´jer-ē)	freezing the skin with liquid nitrogen
debridement	(dā-brēd´mon)	removal of nonliving tissue
excision	(ek-sizh´ŭn)	resect, move
incision and drainage		cutting into and leaving open for drainage
irrigation	(ir-i-gā´shŭn)	washing out a cavity
ligation	(lī-gā´shŭn)	tie
pack		tightly pack material into cavity
prepped	(prept)	prepared for a procedure

3.5 Medications

KEY_terms_ The medications that appear in the dictation for this chapter are described below. Study each medication's spelling, pronunciation, and classification.

MEDICATION	PRONUNCIATION	CLASSIFICATION
acyclovir	(ā-sī´klō-vir)	antiviral
Ancef	(an´sef)	antibiotic
aspirin	(as´pi-rin)	analgesic; antipyretic
Bacitracin	(bas-i-trā´sin)	antibiotic
Betadine	(bā´tă-dīn)	antimicrobial
Coumadin	(kū´mă-din)	anticoagulant
E.E.S. (brand of erythromycin)		antibiotic
hydrocortisone	(hī-drō-kōr´ti-sōn)	corticosteroid
Iodoform	(ī-ōd´ō-form)	antimicrobial
Keflex	(kĕf´lĕx)	antibiotic
Kwell	(kwell)	scabicide
lidocaine	(lī´dō-kān)	anesthetic; antiarrhythmic
liquid nitrogen	(nī´trō-jen)	cryotherapeutic agent
Oxy-10	(oxē´ten)	keratolytic
Retin A	(ret´in-ā)	keratolytic
saline	(sā´lēn)	salt solution
tetanus booster	(tet´ă-nŭs)	vaccine
Tylenol #3	(tī´len-ol)	analgesic
Xylocaine	(zī´lō-kān)	anesthetic

3.6 Related Terms

KEY_terms_ The following terms appear in the dictation for this chapter. Study the spelling, pronunciation, and meaning of these terms.

TERM	PRONUNCIATION	MEANING
Ace bandage	(ās)	elastic bandage
copious	(kō´pē-us)	large amount
inflamed	(in´flāmd)	tissue reaction
neonatal	(nē-ō-nā´tăl)	birth to 28 days
presents	(prē´zentz)	appear for examination
sterilely	(ster´il-lē)	free from living organisms
Vicryl suture	(vī´kril)	type of suture material

3.7 Build Your Editing Skills

In this section, you will gain the skills you need to correctly transcribe medical documents.

Selecting the Right Word

The words listed here are often confused in transcription because they sound alike when dictated but have different meanings. Study the words carefully so you will be able to select the correct term according to the context of the dictation.

TERM	MEANING	EXAMPLE
boarder	a person or animal paying a fee for lodging	Our new boarder is a student at the local college.
border	edge; margin	The border of the lesion was inflamed.
sight	ability to see; vision	The sight in the patient's left eye was impaired as a result of the accident.
site	location	The incision site was prepped and draped.
soar	to rise high in the air; float	The plane soared above the clouds.
	to rise to a high level	The patient's desire to walk soared after surgery.
sore	wound	The patient's sore was washed out with saline.
	painful, aching, tender	The abdomen will be sore for a week following the procedure.

Using the Correct Punctuation

Medical transcriptionists apply correct punctuation when preparing medical documents. Review the following punctuation guidelines. (The basic medical transcription guidelines are in Appendix A.)

GUIDELINE

Capitalize races, peoples, religions, and languages, but generally not color designations such as *white* or *black*.

EXAMPLE

The patient is a 5-year-old Caucasian male.

The patient is a 5-month-old white male.

The patient is a 5-week-old black male.

The patient did not speak English.

STYLE TIP

Note that units of time in text are not abbreviated: a 5-year-old patient.

Insert a space between the number and its measurement.

The lesion was 2.0 mm in length.

Use a comma to set off an introductory clause or phrase.

If Dr. Larsen is late, the patients will have to wait.

STYLE TIP

The title of *doctor* is abbreviated when used before a name.

Name _____ Date _____

Exercise 3.1 Building Your Medical Vocabulary

Directions Define the following combining forms.

Term	Definition
1. dermo, dermato	_____
2. erythro	_____
3. maculo	_____
4. papulo	_____
5. vesiculo	_____

Exercise 3.2 Matching Symptoms and Disease Descriptions

Directions Match each word from Column 2 with its definition in Column 1.

Column 1		Column 2
____ **1.** skin eruption caused by mites	**a.**	abscess
____ **2.** overgrowth of scar tissue	**b.**	acne
____ **3.** mole	**c.**	basal cell
____ **4.** lice	**d.**	cellulitis
____ **5.** inflammation of skin and subcutaneous tissue	**e.**	contusion
____ **6.** inflammation of oil glands	**f.**	cyst
____ **7.** oily skin	**g.**	impetigo
____ **8.** wart	**h.**	keloid
____ **9.** fluid-filled sac	**i.**	nevus
____ **10.** skin cancer	**j.**	paronychia
____ **11.** collection of pus	**k.**	pediculosis
____ **12.** contagious infection with pimples and crusting	**l.**	plantar wart
____ **13.** infected hangnail	**m.**	scabies
____ **14.** viral condition on sole of foot	**n.**	seborrhea
____ **15.** bruise	**o.**	verucca

Exercise 3.3 Using the Correct Term

Directions Fill in the blanks by using the following terms.

abrasion	eruption	nodules
analgesics	erythema	papules
antibiotics	indurated	pruritus
blister	laceration	pustules
comedos	macules	vesicles
ecchymosis		

The patient fell off his bicycle and injured his left leg. There is no (**1**)_____

(open cut). The (**2**)_____ (area where the top skin is gone) also shows

(**3**)_____ (redness) and the beginning visible signs of (**4**)_____ (black

and blue). There is no (**5**)_____ (fluid under the skin). The (**6**)_____

(rash) consists of (**7**)_____ (colored spots), (**8**)_____ (raised spots),

(**9**)_____ (fluid-filled pimples), and (**10**)_____ (pimples containing

pus). (**11**)_____ (blackheads) are present. The area is not (**12**)_____

(hard), and there are no (**13**)_____ (knoblike masses). Subjectively, there is

(**14**)_____ (intense itching).

Two prescriptions were given. They were classified as (**15**)_____ (antibacterial

medication, such as Keflex) and (**16**)_____ (pain reliever, such as Tylenol).

Exercise 3.4 Practicing Procedural Terms

Directions Match each procedure in Column 2 to its definition in Column 1.

Column 1	Column 2
_____ 1. specimen checked to see what organism grows	a. anesthetized
_____ 2. wound washed out with saline	b. cauterized
_____ 3. lesion covered with sterile bandage and Ace wrap	c. chemotherapy
_____ 4. tissue cut into with #11 blade	d. cryosurgery
_____ 5. bleeder tied off	e. culture
_____ 6. Xylocaine administered to produce loss of sensation	f. curettaged
_____ 7. abscess pocket scraped of pus	g. drained
_____ 8. Iodoform gauze pushed into the cavity	h. dressing
_____ 9. area cleansed with Betadine	i. incised
_____ 10. tissue frozen with liquid nitrogen	j. irrigated
_____ 11. bleeding of tiny vessels controlled by burning	k. ligated
_____ 12. prescription for Keflex 500 mg	l. packed
_____ 13. pus and sebum extracted	m. prepped

Exercise 3.5 Applying Your Editing Skill

Directions Circle the correct answer in each of the following sentences.

1. Dr. Larsen's son will be a *boarder / border* at the Highland Hills Ski Lodge for the winter.

2. The *boarder / border* of the wound was markedly reddened.

3. This child has a *soar / sore* on the left knee.

4. After being medicated, the patient stated that he could *soar / sore* above the clouds.

5. The surgeon noted the incision *sight / site* with a marking pen.

6. The eye drops will blur the patient's *sight / site*.

7. The patient is a 45-year-old, well-nourished, well-developed *black / Black* female.

8. The physician cleaned *4 cm / 4cm* on the right forearm laceration.

9. When the doctor comes *in / in*, please have her contact the hospital.

10. The physician incised a *2.25cm. / 2.25 cm / 2.25-cm* area of skin.

11. If the pain *persists / persists,* the patient may use a pain reliever.

12. The specimen was *3.5 cm / 3.5cm* in length.

13. The patient is a well-developed, well-nourished *caucasian / Caucasian* female.

14. The patient had numerous purulent *soars / sores* on the left cheek.

15. We need to hire a *spanish / Spanish* interpreter.

HINTS FOR TRANSCRIPTION

Before you begin the transcription for this chapter, be sure you know the following items:

- Enumerating diagnoses
- Keeping units of measure on the same line (for example, 30 mg)
- The pharmaceutical abbreviations in Appendix B
- Use of symbols for units of measurement in Appendix A

MEDICAL DOCUMENT TRANSCRIPTION

You are now ready to transcribe the dictation for Chapter 3.

 The dictation for this chapter is by John Blackburn, MD. Remember to identify each report properly in the upper right corner.

Chapter 3, Item 1
Your Name
Current Date

---

3 TRANSCRIPTION CHECKOFF SHEET

Use the transcription checkoff sheet to record your work and track your progress as a medical transcriptionist.

DOCTOR DICTATING John Blackburn, MD
TYPE OF DICTATION Chart notes, procedure notes, and letters
DATE OF TRANSCRIPTION April 5, 20—

Item Number	Patient	Date Started	Date Completed	Grade/ Number of Errors
3.1	Karen McMillan			
3.2	Letter to Alan McDonald, MD, 6500 Eagle St., Denver, CO 80239-1287 RE: Patricia Smith-Wright			
3.3	David Bondham			
3.4	Ronald Glazier			
3.5	Letter to Alan McDonald, MD, 6500 Eagle St., Denver, CO 80239-1287 RE: Lee Yang			
3.6	Elizabeth Norbak			
3.7	Summer Raintree			
3.8	Hank Rice			
3.9	Nancy Hurr			
3.10	Teresa Bixby			
3.11	Lucas Everson			
3.12	Janet Grossman			

The Respiratory System

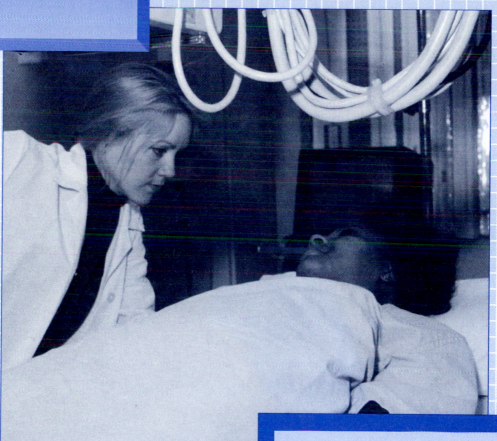

Chest x-rays help assess the condition of the patient's respiratory system. *What medical terms are often used to describe healthy lungs?*

Objectives

After completing this chapter, you will be able to

1. Use correct terms when transcribing medical documents covering respiratory system functions, assessment, conditions, procedures, and medications.

2. Use reference material as needed to transcribe the results of laboratory tests of the respiratory system.

3. Use appropriate terminology when transcribing the results of radiological examinations.

4. Correctly format a letter following appropriate AAMT style guidelines.

4.1 Understanding the Respiratory System

The function of the respiratory system is to exchange oxygen from the air and carbon dioxide from the body cells. This process is known as *respiration*. A *respiration* involves *inspiration*, or inhaling once (taking air into the system), and *expiration*, or exhaling once (letting air out of the system). A person's average respiratory rate is between 8 and 24 times per minute. Control of this rate is accomplished by a person's will, nerves or chemicals, and the use of the muscles between the ribs (intercostal muscles) and the muscle separating the thorax from the abdomen (diaphragm).

The breathing process is accomplished by the following organs (locate each organ on the diagram in Figure 4.1):

Figure 4.1

The Respiratory System

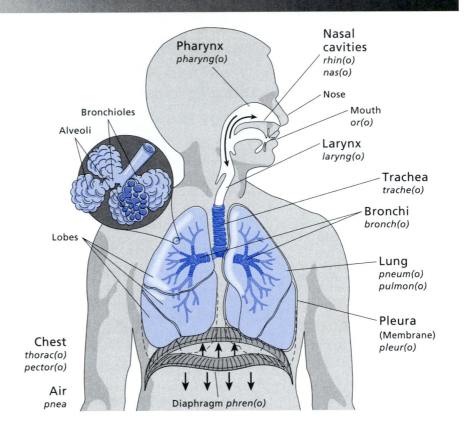

- **Nose** The nose is divided by a cartilage septum into two chambers *(nostrils or nares).* Air enters the nose through the right and/or left nostril *(naris).* The nose, as well as the entire air pathway, is lined with *mucous membrane (mucosa),* which secretes mucus. *Turbinates* are bony projections within the nose. *Paranasal sinuses* surround the nose and secrete mucus that drains into the nasal passageway. (A diagram of the paranasal sinuses is shown in Figure 4.2.) *Adenoids* are a specialized mass of tissue located posteriorly in the nose.

Figure 4.2

The Structures of the
Paranasal Sinuses

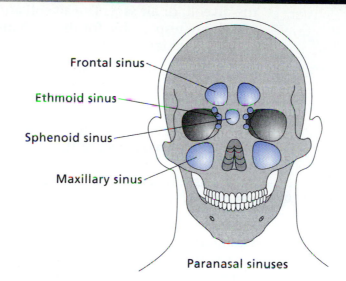

Frontal sinus

Ethmoid sinus

Sphenoid sinus

Maxillary sinus

Paranasal sinuses

- **Mouth** Air, as well as food, enters the mouth. The roof of
  the mouth has landmarks known as the *hard and soft palates*.
  Laterally and posteriorly in the mouth are the specialized
  structures known as the *tonsils*.

- **Pharynx** This organ is commonly called the throat. The
  pharynx is divided into three regions:

  Nasopharynx is the region behind the nose. The eustachian
  tube from the ear opens into the nasopharynx.

  Oropharynx is the region in back of the mouth.

  Laryngopharynx is the region of the voice box, just before
  the branching that separates the air pathway from the food
  pathway. The eustachian tube from the ear opens into the
  nasopharynx.

- **Larynx** This is the organ known as the voice box. It is here that
  a cartilage known as the *epiglottis* prevents food from entering
  the air pathways.

- **Trachea** The trachea, commonly known as the windpipe, is
  located in the midline of the neck and branches as it enters the
  chest region. The trachea is in front of the food pathway. Other
  structures in the neck *(cervical region)* are the lymph nodes,
  which are located laterally and under the chin *(submandibular)*.
  These enlarge when there is localized infection.

- **Bronchi** The main air pathways branch off the trachea,
  forming the right *bronchus* and left *bronchus* (plural—*bronchi*)
  within the lung.

- **Bronchioles** These are the smaller air pathways branching off
  the bronchi and ending in the alveoli.

- **Alveoli** Within the lungs are the branching structures ending in the alveoli, or air sacs. The alveoli and their surrounding blood vessels are responsible for the exchange of gases (oxygen and carbon dioxide).

- **Lungs** The lungs are located in the chest (thorax). They are divided into sections called *lobes*. Each lung is contained within a lining called the *pleura*.

- **Ears** The ears are placed in this system because of their close relationship to diseases of the respiratory system.

4.2 Clinical Assessment

Assessment of the respiratory system includes the head, eyes, ears, nose, throat (HEENT), neck, and lungs. The heart and abdomen are frequently included in the examination, even though the chief complaint refers to the respiratory system.

- **Eyes** The eyes connect to the respiratory system by the tear duct, which opens into the nasal cavity. The conjunctivae should be clear, not reddened, tearing, or mattery.

- **Ears** The eustachian tube connects the nasopharynx and the middle ear; thus an infection that begins as a sore throat may spread and become an earache. The ears should be free of discharge; auditory canals should be clear without cerumen; and the tympanic membranes (TMs) should be flat and pearly gray in color, have good light reflexes, and have normal landmarks.

- **Nose** Nasal drainage should be clear if present. Cloudy or colored drainage indicates an infection, usually connected to the sinuses.

- **Mouth** The oropharynx (mouth and throat) should be moist and without lesions. The tonsils (if present) should not be enlarged.

- **Neck** Cervical (neck) adenopathy usually indicates an infection in the head region.

- **Lungs** Lungs should be clear with good air entry. Breath sounds should be normal without rales, rhonchi, rubs, or wheezes.

Obtaining a history about a cough is very important, since it assists in determining where the problem occurs. The examiner asks if the cough is dry or loose, productive or nonproductive of sputum, and what the nature of the sputum is. The appearance of sputum assists in making a diagnosis. For example, pink-tinged, rusty sputum may indicate bleeding and/or pneumonia; yellowish-green sputum is more common in bronchitis; and copious amounts of watery sputum are common in pulmonary congestion.

The examiner uses observation to assess the amount of oxygen getting into the body tissues: the color of the skin and nails, difficulty with inspiration and expiration, contour and movement of chest, and severity of infections. These might indicate the presence of adenopathy. By palpating the chest, the examiner detects deficient movements of the chest. Percussion and auscultation are used in assessing chest sounds to detect good air entry or diminished air flow (obstruction), consolidation of lung, or the presence of fluid (infiltrate).

4.3 Symptoms and Disease Conditions

KEY_terms_ The following symptoms and disease conditions apply to the respiratory system. Each term on this list is pronounced at the beginning of the dictation for this chapter. Study the list carefully, practicing pronunciation and building word recognition. Be sure you can spell each term correctly.

TERM	PRONUNCIATION	MEANING
adenopathy	(ad-ĕ-nop´ă-thē)	enlargement of lymph nodes (also called _lymphadenopathy_)
asthma	(az´mă)	condition of lungs in which there is narrowing of air pathways, resulting in difficulty breathing
barrel chested		having a rounded (barrel or box car) shape to chest
bronchitis	(brong-kī´tis)	inflammation in the bronchi
bronchospasm	(brong´kō-spazm)	contraction of bronchi, causing narrowing of the lumen (opening)
chronic obstructive pulmonary disease (COPD)		general term for diseases in which forced expiratory flow is slowed
congestion	(kon-jes´chŭn)	accumulation of abnormal amount of fluid or blood
cough	(kawf)	sudden forcing of air from respiratory tract
crackle	(krak´l)	sound in lungs similar to rolling hairs between fingers
croup	(krūp)	noisy, barklike respirations
dysphagia	(dis-fā´jē-ă)	difficulty swallowing
dyspnea	(disp-nē´ă)	difficulty breathing (_dyspnea on exertion_ refers to difficulty breathing during physical activity)
edema	(e-dē´mă)	accumulation of excess fluid in the tissue
emphysema	(em-fi-sē´mă)	abnormal increase in size of air sacs (alveoli)
exacerbation	(eg-zas-er-bā´shŭn)	increase in symptom(s)
exudate	(eks´ū-dāt)	material deposited on tissue as a result of infection
fibrotic	(fī-brot´ik)	referring to tough or strong material

TERM	PRONUNCIATION	MEANING
friction rub	(frik´shŭn)	grating or creaking sound when pleurae rub together
hoarse	(hōrs)	having a rough, harsh voice
hydration	(hī´drā´shŭn)	adequate tissue fluid; not dehydrated
infiltrate	(in-fil´trāt)	accumulation of fluid in tissue
injection	(in-jek´shŭn)	congestion or increase in fluid
low-grade fever		mildly elevated temperature
malaise	(mă-lāz´)	feeling of uneasiness, of being "out-of-sorts"
orthopnea	(ōr-thop-nē´ă)	breathing discomfort when lying flat
otitis media	(ō-tī´tis mē´dē-ă)	inflammation of middle ear
pharyngitis	(far-in-jī´tis)	inflammation of pharynx (throat)
phlegm	(flem)	abnormal amounts of sticky mucus in the mouth and in the throat
pneumonia	(nū-mō´nē-ă)	inflammation of lung tissue
rales	(rahlz)	rattle heard on auscultation of chest
rhinitis	(rī-nī´tis)	inflammation of the nasal mucosa
rhinorrhea	(rī-nō-rē´ă)	runny nose
rhonchi	(rong´kī)	musical pitch heard on auscultation of chest
shotty nodes	(shot´ē-nōdz)	BB-like (very tiny bumps) feeling of lymph nodes
sinusitis	(sī-nŭ-sī´tis)	inflammation of the sinuses
sputum	(spū´tŭm)	material raised from the lungs
suppurative	(sŭp´yŭr-ă-tiv)	forming pus (purulent material)
tachypnea	(tak-ip-nē´a)	increased rate of breathing
tonsillitis	(ton´si-lī´tis)	inflammation of the tonsils
upper respiratory tract infection (URI)		infection of upper air passages, not involving the lungs
wheeze	(hwēz)	whistling or squeaking sound when breathing

4.4 | Laboratory Tests

KEY*terms* Laboratory studies are performed for the diagnosis of many conditions. Tests that are used in the dictation for this chapter are listed below. Refer to Appendix D for detailed explanations.

TERM	PRONUNCIATION	PURPOSE
blood work	(hē-mō-glō´bin)	WBC (white blood count); hemoglobin;
	(dif-er-en´shăl)	differential (PMNs, lymphocytes,
	(lim´fō-sītz)	monocytes, eosinophils, basophils)
	(mon´ō-sītz)	
	(ē-ō-sin´ō-filz)	
	(bā´sō-filz)	
culture		to "grow" a material in order to identify the microorganism; for example, Group A Beta Streptococcus
	(bā´tă strep-tō-kok´ŭs)	
mono test	(mon-ō)	blood test for infectious
	(mon´ō-nū-klē-ō´sis)	mononucleosis

STYLE TIP

WBC is the abbreviation that is preferred for white blood count. Lowercase wbc is used for white blood cells.

4.5 | Radiology Procedures

KEY*terms* The radiology terms that appear in the dictation for this chapter are described below. Study each term's spelling, pronunciation, and meaning so you are prepared for transcription.

Chest x-rays Chest films are generally taken in the PA (*posteroanterior*) view; a lateral view may also be ordered.

Sinus films Sinus films are used to detect normal translucency or opacity (*clouding*).

STYLE TIP

Use lowercase letters and a hyphen for all usages of x-ray.

4.6 Medical and Surgical Procedures

KEY_terms_ The procedural terms that appear in the dictation for this chapter are described below. Study each term's spelling, pronunciation, and meaning so that you are prepared for transcription.

TERM	PRONUNCIATION	MEANING
inhaler	(in-hāl´er)	device used by patients to inhale medications
nebulizer	(neb´yū-līz-er)	device that converts liquid medication to mist/spray for respiratory tract
PE tubes		tiny polyethylene tubes placed in ear for drainage
spirometry	(spī-rom´ĕ-trē)	pulmonary function test (PFT) that determines how well the lungs are functioning and helps determine causes of shortness of breath; includes FVC (forced vital capacity) and FEV1 (forced expiratory volume in one second)
tonsillectomy and adenoidectomy (T&A)	(ton´si-lek´tō-mē) (ad´ē-noy-dek´tō-mē)	excision of tonsils and adenoids
vaporizer	(vā´per-īz-er)	device to add moisture to the air (steamer or humidifier)

4.7 Medications

KEY_terms_ The medications that appear in the dictation for this chapter are described below. Study each medication's spelling, pronunciation, and classification.

TERM	PRONUNCIATION	CLASSIFICATION
albuterol (trade names: Proventil and Ventolin)	(al-byū´ter-ol)	bronchodilator
Augmentin	(aug-ment´in)	antibiotic
Azmacort	(as´mah-kort)	corticosteroid for asthma
Bactrim	(bak´trim)	antibiotic
Bicillin	(bī´sil-in)	antibiotic
Ceftin	(sef´tin)	antibiotic
Pediazole	(pē´dē-ă-zol)	antibiotic
Prednisone	(pred´ni-sōn)	cortisone
Robitussin	(rō-bi-tus´in)	antitussive
Tylenol	(tī´len-ol)	analgesic

4.8 Related Terms

KEY_terms_ The following terms appear in the dictation for this chapter. Study the spelling, pronunciation, and meaning of these terms.

TERM	PRONUNCIATION	MEANING
audible	(ah´da-bul)	able to be heard
bulging	(bul´jing)	swelling
consolidation	(kon-sol´ĕ-dā´shŭn)	condition of becoming solid
cryptic	(krip´tik)	hidden
diffuse	(di-fyūs´)	spread out
discrete	(dis-krēt´)	separate; distinct
extruding	(eks-trūd´ing)	in a position of being pushed out
gaunt	(gont)	thin and bony; emaciated
nocturnal	(nok-ter´năl)	occurring at night
patent	(pā´tent)	open
retraction	(rē-trak´shŭn)	drawing inward
supple	(sŭp´l)	easily moveable

4.9 Build Your Editing Skills

In this section, you will gain the skills you need to correctly transcribe medical documents.

Selecting the Right Word

The words listed here are often confused in transcription because they sound alike when dictated but have different meanings. Study the words carefully so that you will be able to select the correct term according to the context of the dictation.

TERM	MEANING	EXAMPLE
heal	restore to health	The wound should heal in 10 days.
heel	distal end	The patient had a cracked heel on her left foot.
coarse	rough	The doctor used a coarse file to shave the patient's calloused heel.
course	direction	The doctor must decide what course to follow next.
	course of action	The treatment course will be determined after receiving the results of the diagnostic tests.

TERM	MEANING	EXAMPLE
pleural	relating to the serous membrane enveloping the lungs and lining the pleural cavity walls	There was fluid in the pleural cavity.
plural	including more than one	The plural of *diagnosis* is *diagnoses*.

Using the Correct Punctuation

Medical transcriptionists use correct punctuation when preparing medical documents. Review the following punctuation guidelines. (The basic medical transcription guidelines are in Appendix A.)

GUIDELINE	EXAMPLE
There are no plurals in metrics. Spell out the metric measurement if it is not expressed as a technical measurement or if it appears at the start of a sentence.	There were 10 cm of scar tissue present above the patient's pelvic region. The assistant did not know how many millimeters of tape were used Five milligrams was given to the patient.
Hyphenate the elements of a compound adjective that appears before a noun.	The patient was a well-developed male. **but** The male was well developed.
Hyphenate all *self* compounds.	The patient was self-educated.
Form plurals of capitalized abbreviations by adding a lowercase **s**. Pluralize lowercased abbreviations and mixed abbreviations by adding **'s**.	HEENT showed TMs intact. The rbc's will have to be retested. The mEq's were illegible on the lab sheet.

Spelling Correctly

The following words are used in this chapter's dictation. Study their spelling so you can transcribe them correctly without using a reference.

CORRECT SPELLING	EXAMPLE
doubly	The wound was doubly ligated.
sterilely	The operative area was sterilely prepped and draped.

Name _____   Date _____

Exercise 4.1 Building Your Medical Vocabulary

Directions Match each word from Column 2 with its definition in Column 1.

Column 1	Column 2
____ 1. chest	a. broncho
____ 2. voice box	b. dys
____ 3. windpipe	c. laryngo
____ 4. nose	d. oro
____ 5. ear	e. -rrhea
____ 6. eardrum	f. oto
____ 7. throat	g. -phagia
____ 8. mouth	h. pharyngo
____ 9. lung	i. -pnea
____ 10. main branch off windpipe	j. pneumo/pulmono
____ 11. discharge	k. rhino
____ 12. painful	l. -tachy
____ 13. related to swallowing	m. thoraco
____ 14. related to breathing	n. tracheo
____ 15. fast	o. tympano

Exercise 4.2 Matching Symptoms and Disease Descriptions

Directions Match each condition from Column 2 with its description in Column 1.

Column 1	Column 2
____ 1. feeling of unease; "out of sorts"	a. bronchospasm
____ 2. rattle sound to breathing	b. dysphagia
____ 3. difficulty breathing	c. dyspnea
____ 4. contraction of the bronchi	d. exacerbation
____ 5. increase in symptom(s)	e. hoarseness
____ 6. material raised from the lungs	f. malaise
____ 7. rapid breathing	g. orthopnea
____ 8. difficulty swallowing	h. rales
____ 9. harsh, rough sound to voice	i. sputum
____ 10. difficulty breathing when lying flat	j. tachypnea

Exercise 4.3 Using the Correct Term

Directions Fill in the blanks by using the following terms.

adenoids	eustachian tube	paranasal sinuses	thorax
alveoli	larynx	pharynx	tonsils
bronchioles	nares	pleura	trachea
bronchi			

Air enters the mouth or (**1**) _____ (nostrils). It is directed backward into the (**2**) _____ (throat). The air continues down the throat past the region of the (**3**) _____ (voice box) and into the (**4**) _____ (windpipe). This passageway begins the branching system as it enters the (**5**) _____ (chest). The two major branches are the right and left (**6**) _____. The treelike branching continues into the (**7**) _____ (smaller branches) and ends in the (**8**) _____ (air sacs) where the oxygen is exchanged for carbon dioxide. Accessory structures of the respiratory system include the (**9**) _____ (air-filled cavities located in bone surrounding the nose), (**10**) _____ (canal leading from the ear), (**11**) _____ (special tissue in the nasopharynx) and (**12**) _____ (special tissue laterally in the oropharynx), and the (**13**) _____ (lining around the lung).

Exercise 4.4 Building Anatomical Terminology

Directions Build the medical word for each definition.

1. inflammation of the bronchus   _____
2. visual inspection of the bronchi   _____
3. inflammation of the voice box   _____
4. removal of the voice box   _____
5. visual examination of the vocal cords   _____
6. inflammation of the sinuses   _____
7. inflammation of the lining around the lungs   _____
8. inflammation of the lung   _____
9. removal of the lung   _____

Exercise 4.5 Applying Your Editing Skill

Directions Circle the correct answer in each of the following sentences.

1. The *well known / well-known* physician will speak at the conference.
2. The hospital *coarse / course* was uneventful.
3. The patient had a decubitus ulcer on his right *heal / heel*.
4. The surgeon excised *2 cm / 2 cms* from the lesion.
5. The *WBC's / WBCs* dropped from 15,000 to 13,200.
6. After treatment, the wound will *heal / heel* quickly.
7. The patient is *self employed / self-employed*.
8. The *plural / pleural* flap was raised and returned over the bronchial closure.
9. *Coarse / Course* rales were heard through both lungs.
10. Our new physician is *well known / well-known* in the field of pulmonary medicine.
11. How many *mm / millimeters* were necrotic?
12. The surgeon *sterilly / sterilely* cleaned the incision area.
13. The wound was *doublely / doubly* ligated with 2-0 chromic catgut.
14. The *pleural / plural* of *prognosis* is *prognoses*.

Before you begin the transcription for this chapter, be sure you know the following items.

Commonly Dictated Phrases

TMs are pearly gray. TMs are red and bulging. TMs have normal landmarks bilaterally.

Throat is injected with tonsillar exudate.

Neck is supple with adenopathy. Neck has enlarged anterior and posterior cervical lymphadenopathy.

Chest is clear to auscultation throughout; no rales, rhonchi, rubs, or wheezes.

Transcription of Bacterial Infections

Capitalize the name of the genus but not the species. Do not capitalize the plural or adjectival forms.

Culture is positive for Strep (Streptococcus).

Culture is positive for a strep throat infection.

Culture is positive for Group A Beta Streptococcus.

Culture is positive for H. influenzae.

HINTS FOR TRANSCRIPTION

(continued)

Second-page Headings

If a medical document is more than one page, key the word *continued* at the bottom of each page prior to the last page. The second-page heading varies according to the employer's preference but should include pertinent data such as the patient's name, chart number, page number, and date. The continuation pages must have more than one line of dictation and cannot include only the signature line. For transcription purposes in this text, use the following format:

Patient's name   Page 2
(at left margin)   (at right margin)

The second-page heading for a letter does not include the word *continued* and has three items that can be keyed at the left margin as follows:

Addressee
Page 2
Date (then press Enter two or three times before continuing)

MEDICAL DOCUMENT TRANSCRIPTION

You are now ready to transcribe the dictation for Chapter 4.

The dictation for this chapter is by Debra Litman, MD. Remember to identify each report properly in the upper right corner.

Chapter 4, Item 1
Your Name
Current Date

---

4 TRANSCRIPTION CHECKOFF SHEET

Use the transcription checkoff sheet to record your work and track your progress as a medical transcriptionist.

DOCTOR DICTATING Debra Litman, MD
TYPE OF DICTATION Chart notes and letters
DATE OF TRANSCRIPTION April 10, 20—

Item Number	Patient	Date Started	Date Completed	Grade/ Number of Errors
4.1	Ronald Myers			
4.2	Andrea Sandstrom			
4.3	Jordan Adams			
4.4	Letter to Elizabeth Freeman, MD, Otolaryngology Department, 6500 Eagle Street, Denver, CO 80239-1020 RE: Anthony Walters			
4.5	Letter to Janet Sullivan, MD, Department of Pulmonary Medicine, 6500 Eagle Street, Suite 525, Denver, CO 80239-1020 RE: Jack Manly			
4.6	Claudia Stein			
4.7	Leonard Reichart			
4.8	Michael Hite			
4.9	Duane Lofgren			
4.10	Letter to Tomas Berez, MD, 3599 Dexter Street, Denver, CO 80208-2312 RE: Charles Jefferson			

TRANSCRIPTION TEST 1

After the Chapter 4 transcription has been corrected and returned to you for review, you are ready to take Transcription Test 1. Obtain testing information from your instructor.

CHAPTER 5

The Cardiovascular System

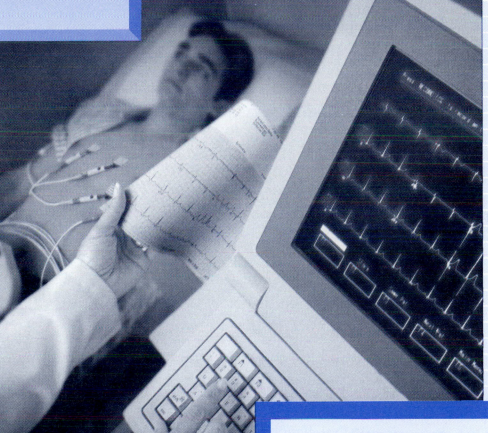

An electrocardiogram (ECG) measures the amount of electrical activity in the patient's heart muscle. *What other procedures are commonly performed to provide information about the heart's health?*

Objectives

After completing this chapter, you will be able to

1. Use correct terms when transcribing medical documents covering cardiovascular system functions, assessment, conditions, procedures, and medications.

2. Use reference material as needed to transcribe the results of electrocardiogram reports and blood tests.

3. Use symbols correctly when transcribing dictation for the cardiovascular system.

4. Apply appropriate AAMT style guidelines to edit and format medical documents.

5.1 Understanding the Cardiovascular System

The cardiovascular system is the body's transportation service. The system includes the blood, the heart, blood vessels, and the lymphatic system. The cardiovascular system's main function is to pump blood to and from the cells of the body. Circulation results in

- **Nutrition** Nutrition is made possible by the cardiovascular system's transportation of glucose, protein, minerals, and fats in the blood to the body cells.

- **Excretion** Excretion is the process by which metabolic wastes are eliminated from the body cells. These wastes are carried away from the body cells during blood circulation.

- **Protection** Protection is provided by transportation of antibodies for resistance to infection.

- **Regulation of body fluids** This regulatory function helps balance the body's temperature.

- **Respiration** Respiration provides for the transportation of oxygen and carbon dioxide.

Blood

Blood has the following components and values:

1. The erythrocytes (red blood cells) contain hemoglobin, which carries oxygen. The normal hemoglobin value is listed as 14 to 16 grams (g) per 100 cubic centimeters (cc) of blood.

2. Leukocytes (white blood cells) assist in fighting infections, respond to allergens, and destroy foreign cells. The normal count of leukocytes in the body is 5000 to 10,000. There are several kinds of white cells, including the polymorphonuclear (PMNs), lymphocytes, monocytes, eosinophils, and basophils.

3. Platelets (thrombocytes) function to clot blood.

4. The plasma (liquid part) transports water, nutrients, hormones, salts, and several kinds of proteins.

Heart

The function of the heart is to pump the blood so it will circulate throughout the body. The heart is located in the mediastinum (middle of the chest). It is a double pump. The right side receives carbon dioxide from the body cells and sends it to the lungs, where it is exchanged for oxygen. Then this oxygen-rich blood returns to the left side of the heart. The left side pumps the blood out to the body cells to deliver the oxygen. Actually, both sides pump at the same time, but the blood goes in different directions and is prevented from flowing backward by *valves*. The heart beats (pumps) 60 to 80 times per minute. Because the heart is a muscle, it requires its own blood supply, which is called the coronary circulation.

Figure 5.1

Flow of Blood
Through the Heart

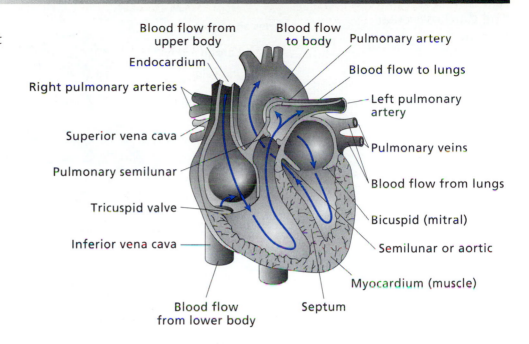

Follow the circulation of blood through the heart shown in Figure 5.1. Blood returns from body cells via the *superior* and *inferior vena cavae,* empties into the right atrium, passes through a valve into the right ventricle, and is pumped to lungs via the *pulmonary arteries.* Oxygenated blood returns via the *pulmonary veins* into the left atrium, passes through the *mitral* valve into the left ventricle, and is pumped out the aorta to the body cells.

Blood Vessels

The blood is transported through a series of vessels, as shown in Figure 5.2 on page 72. Arteries carry blood away from the heart, veins carry blood to the heart, and capillaries surround body cells and exchange oxygen and carbon dioxide, and nutrients and wastes. There are several arterial locations throughout the body where the heartbeat (the pulse) can be felt. Blood pressure is a measure of the amount of force (systole) of the heart pumping the blood through an artery and the relaxation, or filling phase (diastole), of the heart chambers.

Lymphatic System

The lymphatic system is a series of vessels and lymph tissue located throughout the body to assist in transportation as well as filter foreign particles from the blood. The lymph tissue is referred to as nodes, or glands. Tonsils and adenoids are lymph tissue.

The spleen, located in the upper left quadrant of the abdomen and protected by the ribs, manufactures some white blood cells and antibodies as well as salvaging usable iron from the blood stream.

Figure 5.2

The Cardiovascular
System

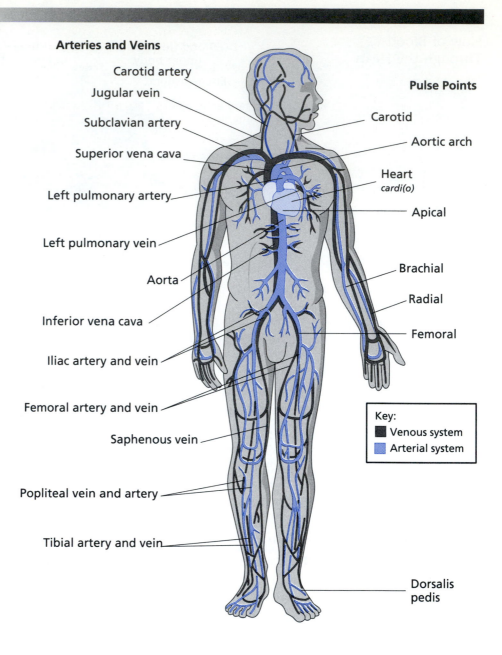

Arteries and Veins

Carotid artery

Jugular vein

Subclavian artery

Superior vena cava

Left pulmonary artery

Left pulmonary vein

Aorta

Inferior vena cava

Iliac artery and vein

Femoral artery and vein

Saphenous vein

Popliteal vein and artery

Tibial artery and vein

Pulse Points

Carotid

Aortic arch

Heart
cardi(o)

Apical

Brachial

Radial

Femoral

Dorsalis
pedis

Key:
Venous system
Arterial system

5.2 Clinical Assessment

The examiner checks heart rate and rhythm. A normal rhythm is referred to as "normal sinus rhythm" that occurs in the sinoatrial (SA) node of the heart. There are several heart sounds as the blood flows through the valves and as they snap shut. The first and second sounds (S1 and S2, respectively) refer to the closing of the mitral and tricuspid valves and then the aortic and pulmonary valves. A third sound (S3) may be heard in children. An S4 is an abnormal sound, as are murmurs, gallops, and rubs. Murmurs may be systolic or diastolic and are described according to loudness in a grading system on a scale of 1 to 6, with 6 being the loudest.

Blood pressure may be considered high when the systolic pressure is consistently more than 140 or the diastolic pressure is more than 90. Normally, there is little difference in the reading if the patient changes position. Fluctuations could indicate a symptom requiring evaluation.

Peripheral pulses should be palpable, equal, and symmetric. They are frequently graded as 2+ *(two plus),* which is a normal grade. There should be no leg, ankle, or pedal (foot) edema.

5.3 Symptoms and Disease Conditions

KEYterms The following symptoms and disease conditions apply to the cardiovascular system. Each term on this list is pronounced at the beginning of the dictation for this chapter. Study the list carefully, practicing pronunciation and building word recognition. Be sure you can spell each term correctly.

TERM	PRONUNCIATION	MEANING
anemia	(ă-nē′mē-ă)	low hemoglobin
angina	(an′ji-nă)	constricting chest pain
arteriosclerotic heart disease (ASHD)	(ar-tēr′ē-ō-skler-ot′ik)	hardening of the coronary arteries
bradycardia	(brād-ē-kar′dē-ă)	slow pulse
bruit	(brū-ē′)	murmur
congestive heart failure (CHF)	(kon-jes′tiv)	increased fluid, especially in lungs, due to poor circulation
coronary artery disease	(kōr′o-nār-ē)	disease affecting blood vessels that supply heart muscle
deep venous thrombosis (DVT)	(vē′nŭs throm-bō′sis)	formation of blood clots in veins
dysrhythmia	(dis-rith′mē-ă)	abnormal heart rhythm; arrhythmia
epistaxis	(ep′i-stak′sis)	nosebleed
fatigue	(fă-tēg′)	feeling of tiredness
gallop	(gal′lop)	fast triple rhythm of heartbeat
hemorrhage	(hem′o-rij)	bleeding not easily stopped; excessive bleeding
hemorrhoids	(hem′ō-roydz)	dilated vein in rectal area
hypercholesterolemia	(hī′per-kō-les′ter-ol-ē′mē-ă)	increased amount of cholesterol (fatty substances) in the blood
hypertension	(hī′per-ten′shŭn)	high blood pressure
murmur	(mer′mer)	abnormal heart sound coming from heart valves

TERM	PRONUNCIATION	MEANING
myocardial infarction (MI)	(mī-ō-kar´dē-ăl in-fark´shŭn)	inadequate blood supply to heart muscle; heart attack
occlusion	(ŏ-klū´zhŭn)	the state of being closed
palpitation	(pal-pi-tā´shŭn)	patient's awareness of heartbeat
peripheral	(pĕ-rif´ĕ-răl)	near the outside; away from heart
rub	(rŭb)	abnormal heart sound (grating or scratchy)
sickle cell anemia	(ă-nē´mē-ă)	inherited abnormality of erythrocytes
stenosis	(ste-nō´sis)	narrowing of blood vessel
tachycardia	(tak´i-kar´dē-ă)	rapid heartbeat
thrombophlebitis	(throm´bō-flĕ-bī´tis)	inflammation of vein due to blood clot
thrombosis	(throm-bō´sis)	blood clot
varicose veins	(vār´i-kōs)	enlarged, tortuous vessel
vascular insufficiency	(vas´kyū-lăr)	inadequate blood vessels

5.4   Laboratory Tests

KEYterms   Laboratory studies are performed for the diagnosis of many conditions. Tests that are used in the dictation for this chapter are listed below. Refer to Appendix D for detailed explanations.

TERM	PRONUNCIATION	PURPOSE
electrolytes	(ē-lek´trō-lītz)	chemicals (in blood) that conduct electricity in tissue
chlorides	(klōr´īds)	
potassium	(pō-tas´ē-ŭm)	
sodium	(sō´dē-ŭm)	
creatinine	(krē-at´i-nēn)	kidney function
complete blood count (CBC)		general physical condition
hemoglobin	(hē-mō-glō´bin)	carrier of oxygen
red blood cell count (RBC)		carrier of oxygen
white blood cell count (WBC) and differential	(dif-er-en´shăl)	indication of infectious process
lipid profile to include cholesterol	(lip´ed) (kō-les´ter-ol)	fatty substances
prothrombin time blood coagulation time (also referred to as INR—international normalized ratio)	(prō-throm´bin) (kō-ag-yū-lā´shŭn)	blood coagulation time

5.5 | Medical and Surgical Procedures

KEY_terms_ The procedural terms that appear in the dictation for this chapter are described below. Study each term's spelling, pronunciation, and meaning so you are prepared for transcription.

TERM	PRONUNCIATION	MEANING
angiogram	(an´jē-ō-gram)	x-ray film of blood vessels after injection of dye
angioplasty	(an´jē-ō-plas-tē)	reconstruction of a vessel
cardiac catheterization	(kath´ĕ-ter-ĭ-zā´shŭn)	insertion of a tube through major vessel into the heart to determine blockage, oxygen content, and pressure
coronary artery bypass graft (CABG)		replacement (graft) of a damaged coronary artery
Doppler ultrasound	(dop´ler)	use of sound waves to detect blood clot
electrocardiogram (ECG or EKG)	(ē-lek-trō-kar´dē-ō-gram)	graphic recording of heart's electrical activity to give information about rhythm, size, and damage to heart muscle; the cycle includes waves referred as _P, Q, R, S,_ and _T_
Holter monitor	(hōl´ter)	continuous recording during normal activities; ambulatory ECG
stress (exercise) ECG (also called treadmill exercise)		graphic recording that evaluates heart's response during physical activity (such as a treadmill)
ventriculogram	(ven-trik´yū-lō-gram)	recording of ventricular activity

STYLE TIP

EKG is an outdated abbreviation for electrocardiogram. The preferred abbreviation is ECG.

KEY *terms*   The medications that appear in the dictation for this chapter are described below. Study each medication's spelling, pronunciation, and classification.

STYLE TIP

Generic, or nonproprietary, names for drugs are not capitalized. A name that is a trademark—also known as the proprietary name or the brand name—is capitalized.

TERM	PRONUNCIATION	CLASSIFICATION
Advil (ibuprofen)	(ī-bū′prō-fen)	NSAID, analgesic
Americaine spray	(ă-mer′kān)	analgesic
aspirin	(as′pi-rin)	analgesic
atenolol	(ă-ten′ōl-ōl)	antihypertensive, antianginal
Ativan	(ăt′ĭ-van)	anxiolytic
Cardizem	(kar′dĭ-zem)	antianginal
Coumadin	(kū′mă-din)	anticoagulant
Demerol	(dem′er-ol)	narcotic analgesic
enalapril	(e-năl′ă-pryl)	antihypertensive
Lanoxin (digoxin)	(lan-ok′sin) (di-jok′sin)	antiarrhythmic
Lasix	(lā′siks)	diuretic
lidocaine (Xylocaine)	(lī′dō-kān) (zī′lō-kān)	anesthetic
Marcaine	(mar′kān)	anesthetic
nitroglycerin	(nī-trō-glis′er-in)	antianginal
Percocet	(per′kō-set)	narcotic analgesic
Procardia	(prō-kar′dē-ă)	antianginal
Vistaril	(viz′tar-yl)	anxiolytic

5.7 Related Terms

KEY_terms_ The following terms appear in the dictation for this chapter. Study the spelling, pronunciation, and meaning of these terms.

TERM	PRONUNCIATION	MEANING
aggravating	(ag´ră-vāt-ing)	make worse
alleviating	(ă-lē´vē-ā´ting)	lessen; relieve
deviates	(dē´vē-āts)	turn aside
extremity	(eks-trem´i-tē)	arm or leg
fingerbreadths	(fin´ger-bredths)	width of a finger; almost an inch
fleeting	(flēt´ing)	passing swiftly
hyperkinesis	(hī´per-ki-nē´sis)	increased muscular movement
inverted	(in-ver´ted)	changed to opposite direction
lightheadedness	(līt-hed´ed-ness)	dizziness
modalities	(mō-dal´i-tēz)	form, method
obliteration	(ob-lit-er-ā´shŭn)	blot out; destroy
ostium	(os´tē-ŭm)	opening
reflexes	(rē´fleks-ez)	involuntary movements
sublingual	(sŭb-ling´gwăl)	under the tongue
TED (thromboembolic disease) stockings		elastic support hose
tremulous	(trem´yū-lŭs)	quivering

5.8 Build Your Editing Skills

In this section, you will gain the skills you need to correctly transcribe medical documents.

Selecting the Right Word

The words listed here are often confused in transcription because they sound alike when dictated but have different meanings. Study the words carefully so you will be able to select the correct term according to the context of the dictation.

TERM	MEANING	EXAMPLE
arrhythmia	loss of rhythm; irregularity of heartbeat	In the heart exam, the doctor detected arrhythmia.
erythema	inflammatory redness of skin	The patient had erythema on both facial cheeks.
discreet	able to keep silent	Please be discreet when talking to the patient's family.
discrete	separate; distinct	There is another discrete lesion on the left forearm.
it's	it is	It's too late to correct the operative report.
its	possession	Place the chart note back in its folder.
mucus	noun, clear secretion of mucous membrane	The doctor will clear the mucus from the patient's mouth.
mucous	adjective, relating to mucus or mucous membrane	The mucous discharge was colorless.
palpation	examination with hands	On palpation of the abdomen, the doctor identified an enlarged spleen.
palpitation	forcible heart pulsation	Heart palpitations increased upon exertion.

Using the Correct Format

Medical transcriptionists apply correct formats when preparing medical documents. Study the guidelines here to learn the rules for the dictation in this chapter. (The basic medical transcription guidelines are in Appendix A.)

GUIDELINE	EXAMPLE
Keep units of measurement on the same line.	The prescription given was for 500 mg t.i.d., #40.
Use lowercase letters with periods for a.m. and p.m.	The appointment was next Tuesday at 10 a.m.
Use roman numerals for cranial nerves, ECG leads, clotting factors, and noncounting listings. Use Arabic numbers with grades and classes.	In patients with a factor VIII or IX level, less than 1% will have severe bleeding. Cranial nerves II-XII were intact. There is a grade 1/6 systolic murmur.

Spelling Correctly

The following words are used in this chapter's dictation. Study their spelling so that you can transcribe them correctly without using a reference.

and/or   The doctor will attend this week's lecture and/or next week's seminar.

cul-de-sac The cul-de-sac in the diverticulum was inspected.

Name _____ Date _____

Exercise 5.1 Building Your Medical Vocabulary

Directions Define the following word forms.

Term	Definition
1. angio or vaso	_____
2. arterio	_____
3. brady	_____
4. cardio	_____
5. cyto	_____
6. -emia	_____
7. erythro	_____
8. hemo or hemato	_____
9. leuko	_____
10. sclero	_____
11. steno	_____
12. tachy	_____
13. thrombo	_____
14. veno or phlebo	_____

Name _____ Date _____

Exercise 5.2 Matching Symptoms and Disease Descriptions

Directions Match each term from Column 2 with its clinical symptom or condition in Column 1.

Column 1	Column 2
____ 1. abnormal sound of heart valves	a. anemia
____ 2. slow pulse	b. bradycardia
____ 3. elevated blood pressure	c. epistaxis
____ 4. varicose vein in rectal area	d. fatigue
____ 5. distended, crooked veins	e. hemorrhoid
____ 6. low hemoglobin	f. hypercholesterolemia
____ 7. blood clot	g. hypertension
____ 8. narrowing of a blood vessel	h. murmur
____ 9. heart attack	i. myocardial infarction
____ 10. inflammation of vessel due to clot	j. occlusion
____ 11. fast heartbeat	k. stenosis
____ 12. nosebleed	l. tachycardia
____ 13. blockage of a vessel	m. thrombophlebitis
____ 14. excessive tiredness	n. thrombosis
____ 15. increased fatty substance in blood	o. varicose vein

Exercise 5.3 Working with Abbreviations

Directions Using Appendix B, provide the meanings of the following abbreviations.

1. ECG _____

2. CBC _____

3. MI _____

4. RBC _____

5. WBC _____

6. BP _____

Exercise 5.4 Building Anatomical Terminology

Directions Match each term in Column 2 with its location in Column 1.

Column 1	Column 2
____ 1. behind the knee	**a.** apical
____ 2. at the heart	**b.** dorsalis pedis
____ 3. at the wrist	**c.** femoral
____ 4. in the groin	**d.** radial
____ 5. in the foot	**e.** popliteal

Exercise 5.5 Locating Vessels

Directions Match the term in Column 2 with its location in Column 1.

Column 1	Column 2
____ 1. main vein in the neck	**a.** aorta
____ 2. vessel carrying blood from heart to lungs	**b.** carotid
____ 3. main artery leaving left ventricle	**c.** femoral
____ 4. vein entering right atrium	**d.** iliac
____ 5. vessel in lower leg	**e.** jugular
____ 6. major vein in thigh region	**f.** pulmonary artery
____ 7. major artery in thigh region	**g.** pulmonary veins
____ 8. main artery in neck	**h.** saphenous
____ 9. vessel branching off the aorta in abdomen	**i.** tibial
____ 10. vessels bringing blood from lungs	**j.** vena cava

Exercise 5.6 Understanding Medical Documents

Directions Using Appendix D, answer the following questions.

| Question | Answer |

Question   **Answer**

1. What is the normal WBC range? _____

2. What condition does the hemoglobin test detect? _____

3. Amylase levels are increased in what disease process? _____

4. Prolonged use of diuretics may lead to deficiency in which electrolyte? _____

5. Dehydration may cause a decrease in which electrolyte? _____

6. What is the term for the rate at which blood will clot? _____ (time)

7. Normal INR is generally maintained at what value? _____

Exercise 5.7 Applying Your Editing Skill

Directions Circle the correct answer in each of the following sentences.

1. We need to be *discreet / discrete* when conversing with patients at the front desk.
2. The patient was advised to have surgery *and-or / and/or* chemotherapy.
3. The staff meeting is at 4 *pm / PM / p.m.* tomorrow.
4. The 4-year-old patient coughed up red-brownish *mucous / mucus*.
5. Return the dictionary to *it's / its* shelf in the doctor's office.
6. Intermittent inversion of P wave was noted in leads *2 and 3 / II and III*.
7. The *cul de sac / cul-de-sac* in the cecum was inflamed.
8. The patient had 4 *discreet / discrete* lesions on his back.
9. The doctor was concerned with the amount of *mucous / mucus* discharged.
10. The patient had infiltrating ductal carcinoma of the right breast, nuclear grade *3 / III.*
11. The patient had localized *arrhythmia / erythema* in the left lower extremity.
12. During the night, the patient noted increased *palpations / palpitations.*
13. On examination, the doctor noted an *arrhythmia / erythema* in the upper extremities.
14. The surgeon's continuous *palpations / palpitations* caused the patient pain.
15. There was a grade *2/6 / II/VI* pansystolic murmur.

HINTS FOR TRANSCRIPTION

Before you begin the transcription for this chapter, be sure you know the following items.

Transcription of Blood Pressure Results

The expression "blood pressure 114 over 82" is transcribed as

>BP 114/82

Spell out the term *blood pressure* if it is used without a measurement:

>Return for recheck of blood pressure.

Transcription of Differential Blood Results

Use percentages: PMNs 75%; lymphocytes 25%.

Spell out *percent* when it is used without a measurement:

>What percent is considered normal?

Use of Symbols

Review the correct use of symbols in these examples:

>The patient had a cough x 2 days.
>
>Medication was changed to 100 mg/hr.
>
>Pulses are 2+.
>
>Next, 2-0 chromic catgut was used.
>
>The laceration was 2.0 x 0.5 cm.
>
>The solution was diluted 1:100.

Terms That Sound Alike

Do not confuse *NSAID* (nonsteroidal anti-inflammatory drug) with the medication Ansid (flurbiprofen, an antiarthritic NSAID).

MEDICAL DOCUMENT TRANSCRIPTION

You are now ready to transcribe the dictation for Chapter 5.

 The dictation for this chapter is by Lynn Solinski, MD, and Lee W. Kim, MD. Use either style of format. Remember to properly identify each report in the upper right corner, as shown here:

>Chapter 5, Item 1
>Your Name
>Current Date

---

5 TRANSCRIPTION CHECKOFF SHEET

Use the transcription checkoff sheet to record your work and track your progress as a medical transcriptionist.

DOCTOR DICTATING Lynn Solinski, MD, and Lee W. Kim, MD

TYPE OF DICTATION Chart notes, letters, and history and physicals

DATE OF TRANSCRIPTION April 12, 20—

Item Number	Patient	Date Started	Date Completed	Grade/ Number of Errors
5.1	Betty Forsman			
5.2	Marietta Henley			
5.3	Renee Eckstrom			
5.4	Donald Eickten			
5.5	Bryant Andres			
5.6	Letter to Merlin Williams, MD, 300 Central Avenue, Lakewood, CO 80134 RE: Alyssa Babcock			
5.7	Letter to Margaret Downing, MD, 6500 Eagle Street, Suite 700, Denver, CO 80239-1700 RE: Derek Wood			
5.8	Trent Wilson			
5.9	Letter to Lisa Swankoski, MD, Ivy Lane Clinic, 1241 Ivy Lane, Denver, CO 80220-1872 RE: Ali Saarken			

CHAPTER

6

The Digestive System

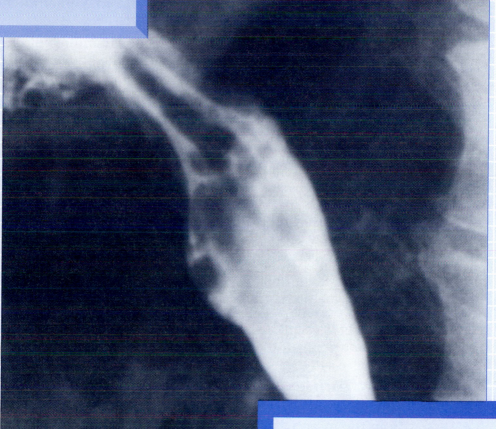

An upper gastrointestinal series is used to assess the digestive system. In this barium swallow procedure, barium sulfate is swallowed and x-rays are taken of the esophagus, stomach, and small intestine. *What abbreviation is commonly used for this procedure?*

Objectives

After completing this chapter, you will be able to

1. Use correct terms when transcribing medical documents covering digestive system functions, assessment, conditions, procedures, and medications.

2. Use reference material to obtain normal lab test values.

3. Apply appropriate AAMT style guidelines to edit and format medical documents.

The digestive system has the following functions:

- **Ingestion** The process of taking nutrients and/or substances and water into the system is known as ingestion.

- **Digestion** This is the breaking down of ingested material into substances that the body can use.

- **Absorption** Absorption is the process of taking nutrients and other substances into the blood stream.

- **Metabolism** The subsequent breakdown and rebuilding of substances so they will be accepted by the body cells is known as metabolism.

- **Elimination** Elimination is getting rid of the waste products that cannot be used by the body cells.

Food nutrients have the following classifications and uses:

Carbohydrates are used for energy.

Proteins build tissues.

Fats are broken down and stored for energy and insulation.

Minerals are needed for metabolism, bone formation, and nerve functioning.

Vitamins are important for metabolism and general overall health maintenance.

Water is essential in the diet to help with transportation of these nutrients in the blood stream.

Gastrointestinal Tract

The digestive (gastrointestinal, or GI) tract is a continuous pathway from the mouth to the anus and includes the following organs:

- **Mouth** This organ is used for ingestion and for the mechanical and chemical breakdown of food.

- **Esophagus** This serves as a pathway for food coming from the mouth.

- **Stomach** Digestion and chemical breakdown of foodstuffs take place in this cavity.

- **Intestine (bowel)** This tubular pathway is where digestive juices, or enzymes, continue the breakdown of food particles and where absorption takes place.

The small intestine is the first part; it consists of the *duodenum, jejunum,* and *ileum.*

The last section of the bowel is the large intestine, or colon, which is divided into sections according to landmarks:

The *cecum* is a C-shaped region in the lower right abdomen.

The *ascending colon* goes up the right side of the abdomen.

The *transverse colon* goes across the upper abdomen.

The *descending colon* goes down the left side of abdomen.

The *sigmoid* is the S-shaped region in the left lower side.

The *rectum* is the last 6 to 8 inches of the colon.

Accessory Organs

In addition to these main organs, there are accessory organs that help with the digestive process. These include the *salivary glands* in the mouth, which add saliva that contains water (for moisture) and digestive enzymes. The *liver* manufactures bile, which is necessary for the metabolism of fats. The *gallbladder* stores the bile. The *pancreas* produces insulin for carbohydrate metabolism and digestive enzymes. The appendix is a structure off the cecum; it has no function.

6.2 Anatomical Landmarks

The following terms apply to the digestive anatomical structure:

- **Abdomen** is the region between the diaphragm and the pelvis (between the hip bones). The abdomen can be divided into quadrants as a method of locating symptoms: left and right upper quadrants (LUQ and RUQ, respectively) and left and right lower quadrants (LLQ and RLQ, respectively).

- **Epigastrium** is the upper middle region of the abdomen over the stomach (*gastrium*).

- **Upper GI Tract** refers to the stomach and duodenum.

- **Lower GI Tract** is also known as the colon and includes the area from the cecum to the rectum.

- **Peritoneum** is the apronlike membrane lining the abdominal cavity.

Follow the digestive pathway in Figure 6.1 on page 88, noting which organs the substances pass through from the mouth to the anus.

Figure 6.1

The Digestive System

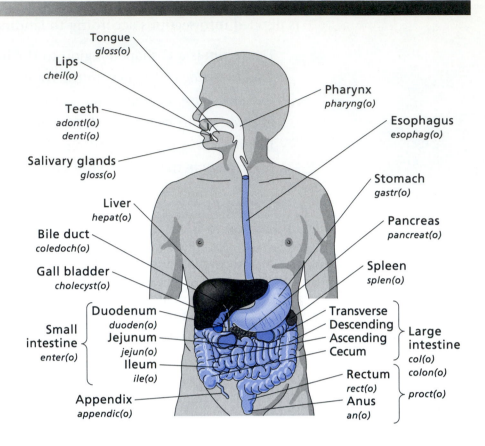

Tongue
gloss(o)

Lips
cheil(o)

Teeth
adontl(o)
denti(o)

Salivary glands
gloss(o)

Liver
hepat(o)

Bile duct
coledoch(o)

Gall bladder
cholecyst(o)

Small intestine
enter(o)

Duodenum
duoden(o)

Jejunum
jejun(o)

Ileum
ile(o)

Appendix
appendic(o)

Pharynx
pharyng(o)

Esophagus
esophag(o)

Stomach
gastr(o)

Pancreas
pancreat(o)

Spleen
splen(o)

Transverse
Descending
Ascending
Cecum

Large intestine
col(o)
colon(o)
proct(o)

Rectum
rect(o)

Anus
an(o)

6.3 Clinical Assessment

An examination of the mouth includes teeth, tongue, mucous membranes, and breath.

The patient's history related to the esophagus and stomach includes symptoms of appetite, nausea, vomiting, pain (where, when, how long, and its character), food intolerance, flatulence, and heartburn.

Symptoms that relate to the intestine include pain, constipation, diarrhea, and bleeding.

A visual examination would include palpation to note tenderness, rigidity, organ enlargement, or masses. Auscultation is used mainly to detect whether or not bowel sounds are present.

Stool (*feces, BM*) is normally brown in color because of the by-products of the digestive process. The anatomy of the intestine gives stool its characteristic shape and size.

6.4 Symptoms and Disease Conditions

KEY *terms* The following symptoms and disease conditions apply to the digestive system. Each term on this list is pronounced at the beginning of the dictation for this chapter. Study the list carefully, practicing pronunciation and building word recognition. Be sure you can spell each term correctly.

TERM	PRONUNCIATION	MEANING
alcoholism	(al´kō-hol-izm)	chronic, excessive drinking of alcohol
anorexia	(an-ō-rek´sē-ă)	diminished appetite
appendicitis	(ă-pen-di-sī´tis)	inflammation of appendix
belch	(belsh)	burp
cholecystitis	(kō´lē-sis-tī´tis)	inflammation of gallbladder
cholelithiasis	(kō´lē-li-thī´ă-sis)	stones in the gallbladder
cirrhosis	(sir-rō´sis)	progressive liver disease
clay-colored stool		no color to the stools
colic	(kol´ik)	spasmodic abdominal pain (adjective—colicky)
constipation	(kon-sti-pā´shŭn)	infrequent hard, dry stool
diarrhea	(dī-ă-rē´ă)	frequent watery or nonformed stool
diverticulum	(dī-ver-tik´yū-lŭm)	pouch in the intestine
dyspepsia	(dis-pep´sē-ă)	indigestion
dysphagia	(dis-fā´jē-ă)	difficulty swallowing
emesis	(em´ĕ-sis)	vomiting
flatulence/flatus	(flat´yū-lens, flā´tŭs)	excessive gas in GI tract
gastritis	(gas-trī´tis)	inflammation of stomach
gastroenteritis	(gas´trō-en-ter-ī´tis)	inflammation of stomach and intestine
hematemesis	(hē-mă-tem´ĕ-sis)	vomiting blood
hematochezia	(hē´mă-tō-kē´zē-ă)	bloody stools
hepatitis	(hep-ă-tī´tis)	inflammation of liver
hernia	(her´nē-ă)	protrusion of an organ
hiatal hernia	(hī-ā´tăl)	protrusion of part of stomach through diaphragm
hypokalemia	(hī´pō-ka-lē´mē-ă)	decreased potassium in blood
icterus	(ik´ter-ŭs)	jaundice; yellowish color to skin or eyes
ileus	(il´ē-ŭs)	bowel obstruction
melena	(me-lē´nă)	dark, tarry stools
pancreatitis	(pan´krē-ă-tī´tis)	inflammation of pancreas
polyp	(pol´ip)	projecting tissue mass
reflux	(rē´flŭks)	backward flow
thrush	(thrŭsh)	fungal or yeast infection of mouth tissue, frequently occurring after treatment with antibiotics
ulcer	(ŭl´ser)	open sore (*Use a medical dictionary to review the different kinds of ulcers.*)

6.5 Laboratory Tests

KEY_terms_ There are many tests included in a chemistry (chem) profile. Some of the more common ones include the following. Refer to Appendix D for detailed explanations.

TERM	PRONUNCIATION
alkaline phosphatase	(al´kă-lĭn fos´fă-tās)
amylase	(am´il-ās)
bilirubin	(bil-i-rū´bin)
blood lipids (fats) 　cholesterol, including total, 　HDL, LDL, and ratio of total 　to HDL	(kō-les´ter-ol)
triglycerides	(trī-glis´er-īds)
BUN (blood urea nitrogen)	(yū-rē´ă)
calcium	
CBC	
creatinine	(krē-at´i-nēn)
electrolytes (sodium, potassium, 　chloride, and CO_2)	

STYLE TIP

If the equipment you are using does not allow for subscripts, place the characters on the same line: CO2.

glucose	(glū´kōs)
SGOT/AST	

A stool test for the digestive system is the hemoccult (guaiac—gwī´ak) test, which checks for blood in the stool specimen.

6.6 Radiology Procedures

KEY_terms_ The radiology terms that appear in the dictation for this chapter are described below. Study each term's spelling, pronunciation, and purpose so you are prepared for transcription.

TERM	PRONUNCIATION	PURPOSE
barium enema	(ba´rē-ŭm en´ĕ-mă)	documents presence of colon disease
flat plate of abdomen		evaluates suspected blockage or perforation of intestine (no contrast material or dye is used)
upper gastrointestinal (upper GI series or UGI)		outlines the upper digestive tract for diseases such as ulcers, may include a barium swallow to examine the esophagus and/or a small bowel follow-through to examine the jejunum and ileum

6.7 Medical and Surgical Procedures

KEY *terms* The procedural terms that appear in the dictation for this chapter are described below. Study each term's spelling, pronunciation, and meaning so you are prepared for transcription.

TERM	PRONUNCIATION	MEANING
appendectomy	(ap-pen-dek´tō-mē)	removal of appendix
cholecystectomy	(kō´lē-sis-tek´tō-mē)	removal of the gallbladder
colonoscopy	(kō-lon-os´kō-pē)	visualization of the colon with a scope instrument
endoscopy	(en-dos´kŏ-pē)	general term for visualization using scope
flexible sigmoidoscopy	(sig´moy-dos´kō-pē)	visualization of the sigmoid using flexible scope
gastric bypass		rerouting pathway to bypass some of the stomach region, commonly done by stapling part of stomach
gastric resection	(gas´trik rē-sek´shŭn)	removal of part of stomach
gastroscopy	(gas-tros´kō-pē)	visualization of stomach using scope
laparoscopy	(lap-ă-ros´kō-pē)	visualization with fiberoptic instrument through the abdominal wall via tiny incision
laparotomy	(lap-ă-rot´ō-mē)	incision through the abdominal wall
ultrasound	(ŭl´tră-sownd)	imaging using sound waves to detect liquid or solid mass or tissue

6.8 Medications

KEYterms The medications that appear in the dictation for this chapter are decribed below. Study each medication's spelling, pronunciation, and classification.

TERM	PRONUNCIATION	CLASSIFICATION
chlorpheniramine	(klōr-fĕn-ir´ă-mēn)	decongestant
K-Dur	(k´dur)	potassium supplement
Lipitor	(lip´ĭ-tor)	hypolipidemic
Lomotil	(lō-mō´til)	antidiarrheal
Maalox	(mā´lox)	antacid
Metamucil	(met´ă-mū-sil)	laxative
Milk of Magnesia	(mag-nē´zhŭh)	laxative
Motrin	(mō´trin)	analgesic
Mylanta	(mī-lan´ta)	antacid
Prilosec	(pril´ō-sik)	antiulcer
Tagamet	(tāg´ă-met)	antiulcer
Toradol	(tor´ă-dol)	analgesic
Zantac	(zan´tak)	antiulcer

6.9 Related Terms

KEYterms The following terms appear in the dictation for this chapter. Study the spelling, pronunciation, and meaning of these terms.

TERM	PRONUNCIATION	MEANING
antispasmodic	(an´tē-spaz-mod´ik)	able to decrease or stop spasms or cramps
claustrophobia	(klaw-strō-fō´bē-ă)	morbid fear of confinement
costovertebral angle	(kos-tō-ver´tĕ-brăl)	area where ribs meet vertebrae and the kidneys are located
digital	(dij´i-tăl)	relating to fingers or toes
GI cocktail		blend of antacid and anesthetic
nonsteroidal	(non-stēr´oy-dăl)	containing no cortisone medication
normocephalic	(nōr´mō-se-fal´ik)	normal-sized head
occult	(ŏ-kŭlt´)	hidden
retroflexed	(re´trō-flekst)	bent backward
scleral	(sklēr´ăl)	pertaining to white portion of eye
screening		testing
sessile	(ses´il)	having a broad base

6.10 Build Your Editing Skills

In this section, you will gain the skills you need to correctly transcribe medical documents.

Selecting the Right Word

The words listed here are often confused in transcription because they sound alike when dictated but have different meanings. Study the words carefully so you will be able to select the correct term according to the context of the dictation.

TERM	MEANING	EXAMPLE
loose	not firmly fastened nor fixed	You need to loosen the screw before turning it. The patient had loose bowels from the medication.
lose	unable to find	Do not lose your credential papers because they are needed for your personnel file.
palate	roof of the mouth	The patient burned his palate on hot coffee.
pallet	temporary bed or portable platform	The kindergarten students were told to place their nap pallets on the floor of the gym.
reflex	automatic or involuntary response; bent back	The patient's reflexes failed during the exam.
reflux	flowing back	After eating spicy foods, the patient was bothered with reflux and continually burped.
than	comparative; used to express difference	Dr. Larsen is shorter than Dr. Newman.
then	at that time	First we must clean the wound area; then we apply the anesthetic ointment.

Using the Correct Punctuation

Medical transcriptionists use correct punctuation when preparing medical documents. Review the following punctuation guidelines. (The basic medical transcription guidelines are in Appendix A.)

GUIDELINE

Do **not** capitalize undesignated rooms (such as operating room), medical specialties, or variations of specialties. Capitalize designated rooms and medical specialties used before names as titles.

Spell out abbreviations in full in medical documents for the diagnosis, conclusion, or procedural/operative title. Nondisease-related abbreviations can be abbreviated.

EXAMPLE

The patient was sent to the operating room at 3 p.m.
Please refer the patient to oncology.
Dr. Nue is in Operating Suite C.
Refer the patient to Cardiologist John Wu.

DIAGNOSIS: Chronic obstructive pulmonary disease.

OPERATION: Excision of two 5-cm benign lesions, back of neck.

STYLE TIP

Spell out one of two adjacent numbers for clarity: two 5-cm benign lesions.

Name _____ Date _____

Exercise 6.1 Building Your Medical Vocabulary

Directions Define the following word forms.

TERM	DEFINITION
1. cholecysto	_____
2. colo	_____
3. duodeno	_____
4. entero	_____
5. esophago	_____
6. gastro	_____
7. hepato	_____
8. ileo	_____
9. laparo	_____
10. litho	_____
11. pancreato	_____
12. -phagia	_____
13. pharyngo	_____
14. procto	_____

Exercise 6.2 Building Words

Directions Provide the medical terms for inflammations involving the following organs.

INFLAMMATION	TERM
1. stomach	_____
2. appendix	_____
3. gallbladder	_____
4. esophagus	_____
5. throat	_____
6. pancreas	_____
7. liver	_____
8. small intestine	_____
9. mouth	_____
10. large intestine	_____

Exercise 6.3 Applying Your Knowledge

Directions Circle the correct term in the following statements.

1. Inflammation of the colon is *choleitis / colitis*.

2. Indigestion is *dyspepsia / dysphagia*.

3. Visualization of the lowest part of the GI tract is *pancreatoscopy / proctoscopy*.

4. Incision into the abdominal wall is *laparoscopy / laparotomy*.

5. The condition of having gallstones is *cholelithiasis / cololithiasis*.

6. Visualization of the stomach is *gastroscope / gastroscopy*.

7. Making a new opening into the small intestine is *ileostomy / sigmoidostomy*.

8. Cancer of the large intestine may result in *colostomy / ileostomy*.

9. A gastrojejunostomy refers to removal of the *duodenum / stomach*.

10. The placement of a permanent feeding tube is a *gastrostomy / gastrotomy*.

11. The patient will take *enteric- / interic-* coated aspirin.

12. Thrush may cause *hepatitis / pharyngitis*.

Exercise 6.4 Matching Symptoms and Disease Descriptions

Directions Match the sympton or disease in Column 2 with the definition in Column 1.

Column 1	Column 2
____ 1. feeling of general discomfort	a. anorexia
____ 2. bowel obstruction	b. cholelithiasis
____ 3. vomiting	c. colic
____ 4. tightening or narrowing	d. dysphagia
____ 5. loss of appetite	e. emesis
____ 6. jaundice	f. hematemesis
____ 7. projecting tissue mass	g. hematochezia
____ 8. vomiting blood	h. icterus
____ 9. open sore	i. ileus
____ 10. abdominal cramps	j. malaise
____ 11. gallstones	k. melena
____ 12. dark-colored stools	l. polyp
____ 13. difficulty swallowing	m. stricture
____ 14. bloody stools	n. ulcer

Exercise 6.5 Understanding Medical Documents

Directions Using Appendix D, circle the correct term in the following statements.

1. Liver disease may be monitored by the *alkaline phosphatase / amylase* test.

2. Pancreatic conditions may be evaluated by the *amylase / creatinine* test.

3. A newborn's bilirubin of 15 is *abnormal / normal*.

4. A cholesterol reading of 200 is considered *above / below / within* normal range.

5. Liver damage due to drug toxicity could be determined by the *transaminase / uric acid* test.

Exercise 6.6 Applying Your Editing Skills

Directions Circle the correct term in the following sentences.

1. FINAL DIAGNOSIS: *ASHD / Arteriosclerotic heart disease.*

2. Antacids did not help the patient's esophageal *reflex / reflux.*

3. The patient left *operating room B / Operating Room B* in good condition.

4. PROCEDURE: Stress *ECG / Electrocardiogram.*

5. After tickling of the palm, the doctor noted the patient's palmar *reflex / reflux.*

6. In examining the 4 extremities, the doctor found systolic BP 30–40 mmHg higher in the upper extremities *than / then* in the lower extremities.

7. The doctor needed a new briefcase lock so that she did not *loose / lose* her documents.

8. The small hammer was used on the knee to test the patient's *reflex / reflux.*

9. The HEENT exam showed several white pustules on the patient's *palate / pallet.*

10. After the patient left the *operating room / Operating Room,* he was transferred to *Recovery Room 2 / recovery room 2.*

11. *Than / Then* 2 hours later, he was moved to a room on the fourth floor.

12. The doctor was sent to *cardiology / Cardiology.* She spoke with *Cardiologist / cardiologist* Sue Brown.

HINTS FOR TRANSCRIPTION

Before you begin the transcription for this chapter, be sure you know the following items.

Commonly Dictated Phrases

The abdomen was soft, flat, and nontender without rebound, masses, rigidity, or organomegaly.

Bowel sounds are normal (active).

The liver, kidneys, and spleen are not palpable (no hepatosplenomegaly).

The rectal exam is negative with good sphincter tone, without fissures or hemorrhoids.

Stool is guaiac negative.

Review Capitalization Usage

For allergies:

The patient was ALLERGIC TO PENICILLIN.

For trade or brand names:

The patient was given Maalox with relief of symptoms.

For races, religions, and languages:

The patient was a well-developed, well-nourished, non-English-speaking Hispanic male.

MEDICAL DOCUMENT TRANSCRIPTION

You are now ready to transcribe the dictation for Chapter 6.

The dictation for this chapter is by Lynn Solinski, MD, and Debra Litman, MD. Remember to properly identify each report in the upper right corner.

> Chapter 6, Item 1
> Your Name
> Current Date

6 TRANSCRIPTION CHECKOFF SHEET

Use the transcription checkoff sheet to record your work and track your progress as a medical transcriptionist.

DOCTOR DICTATING Lynn Solinski, MD, and Debra Litman, MD

TYPE OF DICTATION Chart notes, letter, consultation, procedure notes, and x-ray report

DATE OF TRANSCRIPTION April 15, 20—

Item Number	Patient	Date Started	Date Completed	Grade/ Number of Errors
6.1	Julie Kurland			
6.2	Jeanne Raymond			
6.3	Letter to Lia Luez, MD, Department of Gastroenterology and Rectal Surgery, Eagle Medical Center, 6450 Eagle Street, Denver, CO 80239-7251 RE: Cecil Razido			
6.4	Carol Gregg			
6.5	Laura Eagan			
6.6	Brian Bruder			
6.7	Brian Bruder			
6.8	Harriet Myers			
6.9	Lynn Kelly			
6.10	Edwina Forrester			
6.11	Bruce Noreen			

CHAPTER 7

The Endocrine System

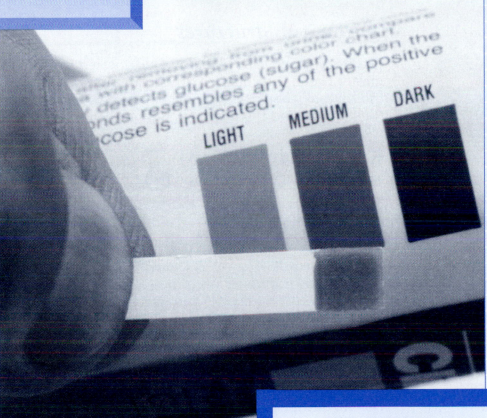

Patients with diabetes mellitus must monitor their glucose level. *What tests and medications are commonly associated with this condition?*

Objectives

After completing this chapter, you will be able to

1. Use correct terms when transcribing medical documents covering endocrine system functions, assessment, conditions, procedures, and medications.
2. Briefly discuss common symptoms of diabetes, hypothyroidism, and hyperthyroidism.
3. Use a reference manual for questionable punctuation, capitalization, or grammar when transcribing.
4. Apply appropriate AAMT style guidelines to edit and format medical documents.

The function of the endocrine system is to produce *hormones*. Hormones are chemicals that regulate the body's activities. They are sent directly into the blood stream and circulated throughout the body. These hormones are interrelated, and their effects overlap. The endocrine system and the nervous system work together to regulate body processes—the first producing long-term effects; the other producing short-term action.

Anatomical Structures

- **Pituitary gland** The *pituitary gland*, located in the head, is the master gland. It regulates many organs and other glands, such as the thyroid gland, the reproductive glands, the adrenal glands, the kidneys, and the uterus, as well as the general functioning of the body.

- **Thyroid gland** The *thyroid gland* is located in the neck around the trachea. Its main function is to regulate the body's metabolism.

- **Parathyroid glands** These glands are located on the thyroid, and their hormones affect the body's use of calcium.

- **Adrenal glands** The *adrenal glands* are located on top of the kidneys. The hormones from these glands respond in times of physiologic stress (disease) and affect kidney function and sexual development.

- **Islets of Langerhans** Within the pancreas, the islets produce insulin, which helps the body's cells accept glucose.

- **Ovaries and testes** The *ovaries* and *testes* are also part of this system, but their functions are discussed in Chapter 9, which covers the reproductive system.

Hormones

A brief summary of some common hormones is shown here. See Figures 7.1 and 7.2.

GLAND	HORMONE	EFFECT
pituitary	thyrotrophin (TSH)	thyroid gland
	adrenocorticotrophin	adrenals
thyroid	thyroxine (T3 and T4)	body's metabolism
parathyroids	parathormone	use of calcium
adrenals	cortisone	physiologic stress
	epinephrine	physiologic stress
islets of Langerhans	insulin	use of glucose
testes	testosterone	male sex features
ovaries	estrogen	female sex features
	progesterone	menstrual cycle

Figure 7.1

Male Endocrine System

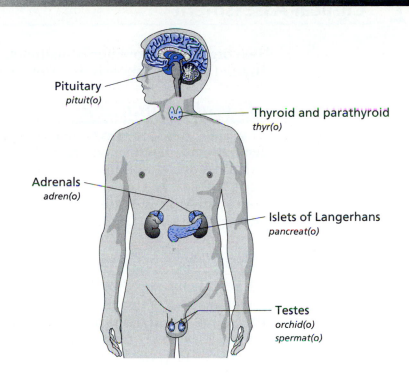

Pituitary
pituit(o)

Thyroid and parathyroid
thyr(o)

Adrenals
adren(o)

Islets of Langerhans
pancreat(o)

Testes
orchid(o)
spermat(o)

Figure 7.2

Female Endocrine System

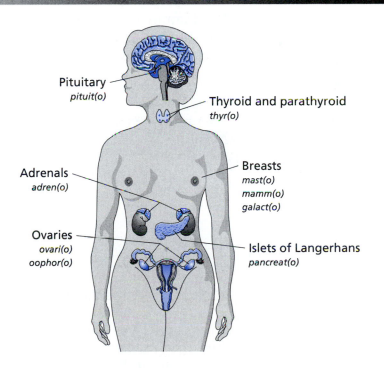

Pituitary
pituit(o)

Thyroid and parathyroid
thyr(o)

Adrenals
adren(o)

Breasts
mast(o)
mamm(o)
galact(o)

Ovaries
ovari(o)
oophor(o)

Islets of Langerhans
pancreat(o)

Two organs that commonly malfunction in this system are the thyroid and the pancreas (islets of Langerhans).

Thyroid Conditions

Thyroid conditions affect the thinking process, energy levels, body temperature, digestive and reproductive processes, and eyes. The examiner asks questions about the thinking process, tiredness, excessive energy, excessive sweating, excessive weight gain or loss, constipation or diarrhea, sensation of being too hot or always cold, tremor, tachycardia, and nervousness.

Diabetes

Diabetes is the body's inability to properly metabolize glucose. This condition affects the entire body, including the kidneys, the nerves (including vision), and the cardiovascular system, especially circulation of the lower extremities.

When the onset of diabetes is in childhood, it is classified as juvenile diabetes (type I) and may be insulin-dependent (IDDM) or noninsulin-dependent (NIDDM) diabetes mellitus. When the onset is later in life, it is classified as diabetes mellitus, adult onset (type II). Generally type II is noninsulin dependent (NIDDM) and is controlled through diet and exercise. If medication becomes necessary, oral medication is preferred rather than insulin injections.

The examiner asks questions about excessive sweating, increased thirst, increased urination, weight gain or loss, visual changes, and changes in sensation (nerve damage).

STYLE TIP

The types of diabetes are indicated by capital Roman Numerals (I, II). The word *type* is lowercase.

7.3   Symptoms and Disease Conditions

KEYterms   The following symptoms and disease conditions apply to the endocrine system. Each term on this list is pronounced at the beginning of the dictation for this chapter. Study the list carefully, practicing pronunciation and building word recognition. Be sure that you can spell each term correctly.

TERM	PRONUNCIATION	MEANING
diabetes mellitus	(dī-ă-bē´tēz mel´ĭ-tus)	inadequate glucose metabolism
type I		juvenile onset
type II		adult onset
gestational		pregnancy related
euthyroid	(yū-thī´royd)	normally functioning thyroid gland
exophthalmos or	(ek-sof-thal´mos)	bulging eyes
exophthalmus		
glycosuria	(glī´kō-sū´rē-ă)	glucose (sugar) in the urine
goiter	(goy´ter)	enlargement of thyroid gland
Graves' disease	(grāvz)	overactive thyroid characterized by toxic goiter
hyperglycemia	(hī´per-glī-sē´mē-ă)	too much glucose in the blood; high blood sugar
hyperthyroidism	(hī-per-thī´royd-izm)	excessive functioning activity of the thyroid
hypoglycemia	(hī´pō-glī-sē´mē-ă)	too little glucose in blood; low blood sugar
hypothyroidism	(hī-pō-thī´royd-izm)	deficiency of thyroid function
nephropathy	(ne-frop´ă-thē)	kidney disease
neuropathy	(nū-rop-ă-thē)	disease involving nerves
polydipsia	(pol-ē-dip´sē-ă)	increased thirst
polyphagia	(pol-ē-fā´jē-ă)	increased appetite
polyuria	(pol-ē-yū´rē-ă)	excessive urination
proteinuria	(prō-tē-nū´rē-ă)	protein in urine
stasis ulcer	(stā´sis)	ulcer due to poor blood flow
thyrotoxicosis	(thī´rō-tok-si-kō´sis)	extreme overactivity of thyroid gland

7.4   Laboratory Tests

KEY_terms_   Laboratory studies that are used in the dictation for this chapter are listed below. Refer to Appendix D for detailed explanations.

Diabetes

TERM	DEFINITION
blood sugar	
fasting (FBS)	fasting for 8 hours
postprandial (pp) (post-pran´dē-ăl)	2 hours after eating
random	at any time
hemoglobin A1c (glycosylated)	estimates glucose control over the preceding 3 months
glucometer (Accu-Chek™)	home blood glucose monitoring kit
BUN (blood urea nitrogen)	kidney involvement
oral glucose tolerance test	diagnostic

TERM	DEFINITION
T3, T-4, TSH	thyroid function

7.5 Medical and Surgical Procedures

KEY *terms* The procedural terms that appear in the dictation for this chapter are described below. Study each term's spelling, pronunciation, and meaning so you are prepared for transcription.

TERM	PRONUNCIATION	MEANING
insulin pump implantation		implanted mechanism for insulin administration
pancreatectomy	(pan´krē-ă-tek´tō-mē)	removal of pancreas
radioactive iodine (RAI or I-131)		destruction of thyroid tissue
thyroid scan		imaging for size and shape
thyroidectomy	(thī-roy-dek´tō-mē)	excision of the thyroid

7.6 Medications

KEY *terms* The medications that appear in the dictation for this chapter are described below. Study each medication's spelling, pronunciation, and classification.

TERM	PRONUNCIATION	CLASSIFICATION
Duoderm	(dū´ō-derm)	wound dressing, occlusive
Estraderm	(es´tra-derm)	hormone estrogen
imipramine	(im-ip´ră-mēn)	antidepressant
levothyroxine	(lē´vō-thī-rok´sēn)	hormone
lisinopril	(līs-in´ō-pril)	antihypertensive
Neosporin	(nē-ō-spor´in)	antibiotic
Premarin	(prem´ar-in)	estrogen hormone
PTU (propylthiouracil)	(prō´pil-thī-ō-yū´ră-sil)	thyroid inhibitor
Synthroid	(sin´throyd)	hormone
Zoloft	(zō´loft)	antidepressant

TERM	PRONUNCIATION
Insulin injections:	
regular	
NPH (neutral protamine Hagedorn)	
Humulin	(hyū´mū-lin)
Lente	(len´tē)
Ultralente	(ul´trǎ-len´tē)
Oral antidiabetic agents:	
Micronase	(mī´krō-nās)
(glyburide)	(glī´byū-rĭd)
Glucotrol	(glū´kō-trŏl)
(glipizide)	(glip´i-zīd)
Glucophage	(glū´kō-fāj)
(metaformin)	(met´ǎ-fōrm-in)

7.7 Related Terms

KEY_terms_ The following terms appear in the dictation for this chapter. Study the spelling, pronunciation, and meaning of these terms.

TERM	PRONUNCIATION	MEANING
fluctuate	(flūk´tyū-āt)	to vary
funduscopic	(fŭn´dŭs-skōp-ik)	characterized by visualization of interior of eye
fungal	(fŭng´gǎl)	caused by fungus
intervention	(in-ter-ven´shŭn)	treatment to alter or change course
normotensive	(nōr-mō-ten´siv)	normal blood pressure
scarred	(skard)	replacement of normal tissue by fibrous tissue after an injury
status post	(sta´tŭs) or (stat´ŭs)	condition that has occurred
suboptimal	(sŭb-op´ti-mǎl)	less than desired

7.8 Build Your Editing Skills

In this section, you will gain the skills you need to correctly transcribe medical documents.

Selecting the Right Word

The words listed here are often confused in transcription because they sound alike when dictated but have different meanings. Study the words carefully so that you will be able to select the correct term according to the context of the dictation.

TERM	MEANING	EXAMPLE
continual	occurring frequently, repeated often	There was continual monitoring of the patient's blood sugar during the hospital stay.
continuous	uninterrupted in space, time, or sequence	Continuous pressure was applied to the wound to stop the bleeding.
plain	easy to understand; uncomplicated or unadorned	A plain dressing was applied to the wound.
plane	flat surface	The plane was raised 20 degrees.
sac	part shaped like a pouch, often filled with fluid	The patient had a pustular sac in the right axilla.
sack	container for storing or conveying goods	The patient forgot her shopping sack in the exam room.

Using the Correct Punctuation

Medical transcriptionists use correct punctuation when preparing medical documents. Review the following punctuation guidelines. (The basic medical transcription guidelines are in Appendix A.)

GUIDELINE	EXAMPLE
Use semicolons to separate related independent sentences, independent sentences that contain internal punctuation, independent sentences connected with a coordinate conjunction, and items in a series that already contain commas.	Temperature was 101.2; pulse was 98. If the test is negative, we will proceed with the surgery; or if the test is positive, the surgery will be postponed. We will proceed with the surgery; however, the patient must be aware of the prognosis. The doctor formerly had practices in Los Angeles, California; Tampa, Florida; and Charleston, North Carolina.
Use colons to introduce a series of items, to separate hours and minutes (unless the 24-hour clock is used), and after headings to save space.	The following tests will be performed at the Wilson Lab: glucose tolerance, hemoglobin A1c, creatinine, and total protein. The meeting will begin at 1:30 p.m. Surgery began at 1830. HEENT: Nares are patent. Pharynx is markedly reddened. ABDOMEN: Soft without masses.

Name _____ Date _____

Exercise 7.1 Building Your Medical Vocabulary

Directions Define the following word forms.

Term	Definition
1. dipso	_____
2. endo	_____
3. eu	_____
4. glyco or gluco	_____
5. hyper	_____
6. hypo	_____
7. nephro	_____
8. neuro	_____
9. -phagia	_____
10. poly	_____
11. tachy	_____
12. thyro	_____

Exercise 7.2 Matching Symptoms and Disease Descriptions

Directions Match the symptom or disease in Column 2 with the definition in Column 1.

Column 1	Column 2
____ 1. overactive thyroid	a. diabetes
____ 2. inadequate production of insulin	b. euthyroid
____ 3. fast heartbeat	c. exophthalmos
____ 4. sugar in the urine	d. glycosuria
____ 5. increased thirst	e. goiter
____ 6. kidney disease	f. hyperglycemia
____ 7. excessive urination	g. hypertension
____ 8. normally functioning thyroid	h. hyperthyroidism
____ 9. high blood sugar	i. hypothyroidism
____ 10. bulging eyes	j. nephropathy
____ 11. poorly functioning thyroid	k. polydipsia
____ 12. enlarged thyroid gland	l. polyuria
____ 13. high blood pressure	m. tachycardia

Exercise 7.3 Applying Your Editing Skill

Directions Circle the correct answer in each of the following sentences.

1. The *continual / continuous* ticking of the doctor's watch was making the patient nervous.

2. The level *plain / plane* was changed during the x-ray procedure.

3. The doctor will attend conferences in New York, New York **, / ;** Atlanta, Georgia **, / ;** and Hartford, Connecticut.

4. Please place the patient's sample drugs in a *sac / sack.*

5. The patient should adhere to the following schedule for his new medication **; / :** 2 q.i.d. for 4 days; 2 t.i.d. for 3 days; and then 2 b.i.d. for 10 days.

6. If the surgeon can operate tomorrow, schedule any operating room **, / ;** if he needs to wait until next week, schedule Operating Suite 2B.

7. BP was 120/80 **, / ;** pulse was 88.

8. SKIN **, / :** Mild jaundice.
   HEENT **, / :** Pupils are equal and reactive; fundi appear normal.
   NECK **, / :** Supple.

9. The amniotic *sac / sack* was still intact after 5 hours of active labor.

10. The chief surgeon called the meeting **, / ;** therefore, we will all need to attend it.

11. The emergency surgery took place at *2130 / 21:30* last night.

HINTS FOR TRANSCRIPTION

Before you begin the transcription for this chapter, be sure you know the following items.

Suffixes

Most suffixes, such as *-fold*, *-like*, *-hood*, and *-wise*, are joined directly to the root word without a hyphen.

> The patient needs to return next week in the likelihood that his condition continues.

> Two pouchlike sacs were excised from the left armpit.

Symbols

Use an uppercase **U** when transcribing insulin unit.

> He will take 5 U of regular insulin at night.

Use the zero *(0)* symbol, not the uppercase *(O)* or the lowercase o *(o)*, in numbers.

> The medication was changed to 0.125 mg.

STYLE TIP

Key a zero (0) before a decimal point for clarity: 0.125. Without the zero, the decimal point may not be noticed by the reader.

Lists

A complex string of items such as medications can be in a list format.

1. Premarin 0.625 mg q.d.

2. Synthroid 0.112 mg q.d.

3. Aspirin 5 gr t.i.d.

4. Calcium 600 mg b.i.d.

MEDICAL DOCUMENT TRANSCRIPTION

You are now ready to transcribe the dictation for Chapter 7.

 The dictation for this chapter is by Debra Litman, MD. Remember to properly identify each report in the upper right corner.

> Chapter 7, Item 1
> Your Name
> Current Date

7 TRANSCRIPTION CHECKOFF SHEET

Use the transcription checkoff sheet to record your work and track your progress as a medical transcriptionist.

DOCTOR DICTATING Lynn Solinski, MD
TYPE OF DICTATION Chart notes and letters
DATE OF TRANSCRIPTION April 15, 20—

Item Number	Patient	Date Started	Date Completed	Grade/ Number of Errors
7.1	Russell Hendricks			
7.2	Randy LaMotta			
7.3	Luis Diaz			
7.4	Seymour Teke			
7.5	Letter to Merlin Williams, MD, 300 Central Avenue, Lakewood, CO 80134 RE: Ludwig Grandquist			
7.6	Robert Bias			
7.7	Tashia Bealka			
7.8	Barbara Glickstein			
7.9	Irene Colbert			
7.10	Letter to Roger Capser, MD, Ivy Lane Clinic, 1241 Ivy Lane, Denver, CO 80220-1872 RE: Tia Wytkoff			
7.11	Darla Garske			

TRANSCRIPTION TEST 2

After the Chapter 7 transcription has been corrected and returned to you for review, you are ready to take the second transcription test. Obtain the testing information from your instructor.

CHAPTER 8

The Urinary System

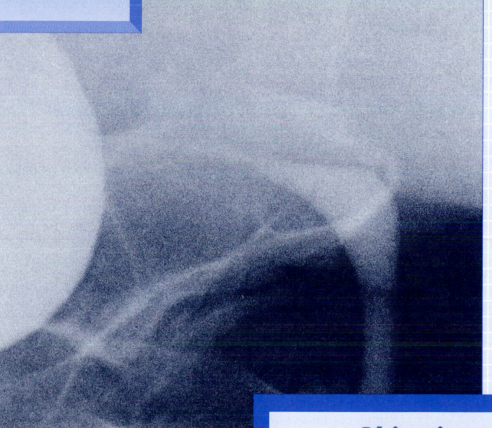

A voiding cystourethrogram (VCUG) is used to assess urinary function. Dye is introduced into the bladder and x-rays are taken of the bladder as well as urethra as patient voids. *What other procedures are used to evaluate the urinary system?*

Objectives

After completing this chapter, you will be able to

1. Use correct terms when transcribing medical documents covering functions, assessment, conditions, procedures, and medications of the urinary system.

2. Use abbreviations correctly when transcribing dictation for the urinary system.

3. Apply appropriate AAMT style guidelines to edit and format medical documents.

8.1 Understanding the Urinary System

The function of the urinary system is to produce urine (waste product of metabolism) and eliminate it from the body. This may be thought of as the process of cleaning or clearing the blood of waste products. Symptoms of malfunction can range from negligible to life-threatening if the kidneys shut down.

The functions of this system include the following:

Regulation of volume and of electrolyte concentration in the body's fluids

Elimination of waste products

Regulation of blood pressure

Urinary Organs

As shown in Figure 8.1, the urinary system has the following organs:

- **Kidneys** There are two kidneys, which are located behind the abdominal organs, against the muscles of the back near the spinal column, and protected somewhat by the ribs. This region is referred to as the *costovertebral angle* (*CVA*). A cushion of fat surrounds the kidneys. The kidneys are bean-shaped and are about 5 inches long and 2 inches wide in an adult. They are made up of many microscopic-sized *nephrons*, which filter materials from the blood. This process results in the formation of waste material known as *urine*. Urine is collected in the basin (pelvis) of the kidney and then drains into the ureters.

- **Ureters** Each kidney has a tube to carry urine to the bladder. Each ureter is pencil-thin and about 10 inches long. The term *flank* refers to the body lateral and posterior area between the bottom ribs and the hip bones. The anatomical region where the ureters and bladder meet is known as the *ureterovesical junction*.

- **Bladder** The urinary bladder is a hollow cavity, anterior to the rectum, and low in the pelvic region (*suprapubic*). The urge to urinate (*void*) occurs when the bladder contains about one-half cup of urine, but the bladder has great stretching ability.

- **Urethra** The tube carrying urine to the outside is the urethra. In the female, the urethra is only about 2 inches long; in the male, it is about 10 inches long as it travels the length of the penis. The male urethra is surrounded by a mass of tissue just below the bladder called the *prostate*. The urethra ends at the *meatus* (orifice), or opening to the outside of the body.

Figure 8.1

The Urinary System

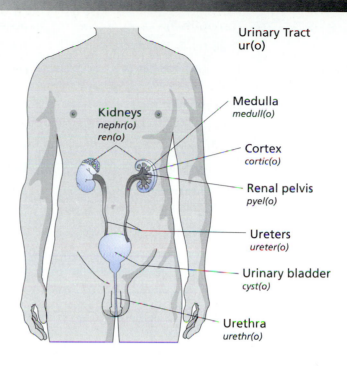

Urinary Tract
ur(o)

Kidneys
nephr(o)
ren(o)

Medulla
medull(o)

Cortex
cortic(o)

Renal pelvis
pyel(o)

Ureters
ureter(o)

Urinary bladder
cyst(o)

Urethra
urethr(o)

8.2 Clinical Assessment

The examiner assesses symptoms relating to urination, hypertension, diabetes, systemic infections, and medications. Examination includes observation of hydration, overall appearance of the body, skin color and turgor, and edema.

Intake and output (*I&O*) is an important consideration in many disease conditions. *Intake* refers to the amount of fluid taken into the body (ingested or parenterally). *Output* refers to the amount of urine, other drainage (nasogastric suction and wound drains), vomitus, and diarrhea expelled from the body. The physician also allows for a certain percentage of loss through respiration and perspiration.

8.3 Symptoms and Disease Conditions

KEY*terms* The following symptoms and disease conditions apply to the urinary system. Each term on this list is pronounced at the beginning of the dictation for this chapter. Study the list carefully, practicing pronunciation and building word recognition. Be sure you can spell each term correctly.

TERM	PRONUNCIATION	MEANING
anuria	(an-yū´rē-ă)	absence of urine
bacteriuria	(bak-tēr-ē-ū´rē-a)	bacteria in urine
benign prostatic hypertrophy, (BPH)	(bē-nīn´pros-tat´ik hī-per´trō-fē)	overgrowth of prostatic tissue (not malignant)
calculus (plural–calculi)	(kal´kyū-lŭs)	stone
colic	(kol´ik)	spasmodic pain, sharp in nature
cystitis	(sis-tī´tis)	inflammation of the bladder
distention	(dis-ten´shŭn)	being stretched
dribbling	(dri´bling)	falling in drops involuntarily
dysuria	(dis-yū´rē-ă)	difficult or painful urination
edema	(e-dē´mă)	excess fluid in tissues
flank		region between ribs and hip
frequency	(frē´kwen-sē)	something that happens at short intervals, as urination
glomerulonephritis	(glō-măr´yū-lō-nef-rī´tis)	inflammation of the filtering mechanism within kidney
hematuria	(hē-mă-tū´rē-ă)	blood in urine
hesitancy	(hez´i-tăn-sē)	involuntary delay in starting the urinary stream
hydronephrosis	(hī´drō-ne-frō´sis)	dilation of kidneys due to obstruction in flow of urine
incontinence	(in-kon´ti-nens)	inability to control urination
lethargy	(leth´ar-jē)	unconsciousness from which one can be aroused, but not without relapses
nephrolithiasis	(nef´rō-li-thī´ă-sis)	the condition of having a kidney stone
nocturia	(nok-tū´rē-ă)	urination at night
oliguria	(ol-i-gū´rē-ă)	scanty urination
proteinuria	(prō-tē-nū´rē-ă)	protein in urine
pyelonephritis	(pī´ĕ-lō-ne-frī´tis)	inflammation of kidney
pyuria	(pī-yū´rē-ă)	pus in urine
reflux	(rē´flŭks)	backflow of urine
residual urine	(rē-zid´yū-ăl)	urine left in bladder after urination
retention	(rē-ten´shŭn)	holding back
stenosis	(ste-nō´sis)	narrowing
stress incontinence		involuntarily expelling of urine during coughing, sneezing, laughing, etc.
ureteritis	(yū-rē-ter-ī´tis)	inflammation of ureter
ureterolithiasis	(yū-rē´ter-ō-li-thī´ă-sis)	stone in ureter
urethritis	(yū-rē-thrī´tis)	inflammation of urethra
urgency	(er´jen-sē)	desire to void immediately
urinary tract infection (UTI)		infection of urinary tract, not including kidneys

8.4 Laboratory Tests

Blood and urine tests are used in the diagnosis of disease processes and to monitor kidney function. Refer to Appendix D for detailed explanations.

TERM	PRONUNCIATION	DEFINITION
alkaline phosphatase	(al′kă-lĭn fos′fă-tās)	blood test
blood urea nitrogen (BUN)	(yū-rē′ă)	blood test
creatinine	(krē-at′i-nēn)	blood or urine test

Urine Test

TERM	PRONUNCIATION	DEFINITION
urine culture (UC) and sensitivity	(kŭl′chŭr)	allowing urine to "grow" to identify an organism, and then testing medications against that organism to identify one that kills it
urinalysis (UA)	(yū-ri-nal′i-sis)	examination of urine
clean-catch/midstream		urinary meatus cleansed prior to obtaining specimen, or the specimen obtained midstream
24-hour urinalysis		collecting all urine voided over 24-hour period

Urinalysis

A great deal of information can be obtrained through the analysis of urine.

Color and clarity Color should be clear. It can vary from almost colorless to dark yellow to tea-colored if it contains blood.

Specific gravity This is normally 1.006 to 1.030. The *pH* indicates acidity or alkalinity, varying from 4.6 to 8.0.

Urine is tested by dipstick (*Clinistix*) and should be negative for *glucose* and *ketones* but may be positive in the diabetic person. Urine that is positive for *protein* or *nitrites* may indicate kidney disease or a heart condition.

Urine is analyzed microscopically. It can normally contain 2 to 5 *red blood cells* (rbc's) per high-powered field (hpf) and fewer than 7 *white blood cells* (wbc's). More white blood cells indicate an infection. Other abnormal findings in the urine include *crystals*, *casts*, and *bacteria*. *Epithelial* cells may be found in urine. *Pus* indicates an infection in the urine. One of the common bacteria found in urine culture is *E. coli* (Escherichia).

STYLE TIP

With lowercase abbreviations such as *wbc* for white blood cells, an apostrophe is used for the plural form: *wbc's*.

8.5   Radiology Procedures

KEYterms   The radiology terms that appear in the dictation for this chapter are described below. Study each term's spelling, pronunciation, and meaning so you are prepared for transcription.

TERM	PRONUNCIATION	MEANING
intravenous pyelogram (IVP)	(ĭn´tră-vē´nŭs pī´el-ō-gram)	intravenous administration of dye (*contrast medium*) and subsequent x-rays (*radiographs*) to see the dye travel through the urinary tract, especially noting the kidneys, ureters, and bladder
plain film of abdomen: kidney, ureter, bladder (KUB)		x-ray without the use of dye; sometimes called a "scout film"
ultrasound	(ŭl´tră-sownd)	imaging using sound waves to detect liquid or solid mass or tissue
voiding cystourethrogram (VCUG)	(sis-tō-yū-reth´rō-gram)	introduction of dye into bladder and subsequent x-rays of bladder as well as urethra as patient voids (urinates)

8.6 Medical and Surgical Procedures

KEY*terms* The procedural terms that appear in the dictation for this chapter are described below. Study each term's spelling, pronunciation, and meaning so you are prepared for transcription.

TERM	PRONUNCIATION	MEANING
catheterization	(kath´ĕ-ter-ĭ-zā´shŭn)	insertion of tube for withdrawal of urine
cystoscopy	(sis-tos´kō-pē)	visual examination of the inside of the bladder
dialysis	(dī-al´ĭ-sis)	artificial means of purifying blood when kidneys are not functioning
dilation or dilatation	(dī-lā´shŭn) (dil-ă-tā´shŭn)	stretching
lithotripsy	(lith´ō-trip-sē)	surgical crushing of stones
nephrectomy	(ne-frek´tō-mē)	removal of kidney
nephrolithotomy	(nef´rō-li-thot´ō-mē)	incision into kidney for removal of stones
transurethral resection of prostate (TUR; TURP)	(trans-yū-rē´thrăl)	entering the urethra for removal of prostate

8.7 Medications

KEY*terms* Sulfa medications are the drugs of choice for infections of the urinary system. Other medications for urinary diseases include antibiotics, antihypertensives, antispasmodics, and analgesics. Study each medication's spelling, pronunciation, and classification.

TERM	PRONUNCIATION	CLASSIFICATION
amoxicillin	(ă-mok-si-sil´in)	antibiotic
Bactrim DS (double strength)	(bak´trim)	antibiotic
Compazine	(komp´ă-zēn)	antiemetic
Keflex	(kĕf´lĕx)	antibiotic
Macrodantin	(mak´rō-dan´tin)	antibiotic
morphine sulfate (MS)	(mōr´fēn sŭl´fāt)	narcotic analgesic
Percocet	(per-kō´set)	narcotic analgesic
potassium chloride	(pō-tas´ē-ŭm klōr´id)	mineral
Pyridium	(pī-rid´ē-ŭm)	analgesic
Septra or Septra DS (double strength)	(sep´tră)	antibiotic

A common IV solution is 5% dextrose (D5) in water or normal saline (salt). It can be prepared in 1-liter (1000 cubic centimeters) amounts.

8.8 Related Terms

KEY *terms* The following terms appear in the dictation for this chapter. Study the spelling, pronunciation, and meaning of these terms.

TERM	PRONUNCIATION	MEANING
accumulation	(a-kum´yū-lā-shŭn)	collection
cerebral palsy	(ser´ē-brăl pawl´zē)	spasms or paralysis due to lesion of brain, usually suffered at birth
configuration	(kon-fig-yū-rā´shŭn)	arrangement or form
contour	(kon´tūr)	outline
dorsal lithotomy position	(dōr´săl li-thot´ō-mē)	lying on the back
epithelial	(ep-i-thē´lē-ăl)	pertaining to outer skin cells constantly being shed; frequently found in urine
hepatosplenomegaly	(hep´ă-tō-splē-nō-meg´ă-lē)	enlargement of liver and spleen
herniorrhaphy	(her´nē-or´ă-fē)	suturing of hernia; hernia repair
lumbosacral	(lŭm´bō-sā´krăl)	relating to vertebral region in lower back adjacent to sacrum (between hip bones)
suppository	(sŭ-poz´i-tōr-ē)	medication given rectally

8.9 Build Your Editing Skills

In this section, you will gain the skills you need to correctly transcribe medical documents.

Selecting the Right Word

The words listed here are often confused in transcription because they sound alike when dictated but have different meanings. Study the words carefully so you will be able to select the correct term according to the context of the dictation.

TERM	MEANING	EXAMPLE
calculus	stone	The IVP showed a calculus.
callus	hard skin; a composite mass of tissue	The callus on the patient's left heel needs to be shaved.

TERM	MEANING	EXAMPLE
healthful	something good for your health or well-being	Healthful foods include most vegetables.
healthy	well, free from disease	In order to be healthy, the patient must follow the doctor's advice.
necrosis	pathologic death of cells, tissue, or organ	There was necrosis surrounding the wound
nephrosis	disease of the kidney	Because of obvious renal failure, the diagnosis was nephrosis.
prostate	chestnut-shaped gland surrounding the begining of the male urethra	The patient will have surgery on his prostate.
prostrate	lying full-length face down; oversome with grief, shock; physically exhausted	The patient was found in a postrate position. The surgeon was prostrate from the 4-hour surgery.

Using the Correct Punctuation

Medical transcriptionists use correct punctuation when preparing medical documents. Preview the following punctuation guidelines. (The basic medical transcription guidelines are in Appendix A.)

GUIDELINE

Hyphenate two-word adjectives such as *follow-up* and *check-up*; combine the two words for nouns, use two separate words for verbs.

Spell out ordinal numbers and single fractions.

EXAMPLE

His follow-up exam will be tomorrow.
We will see her next week for a checkup.
She is to follow up with Dr. Larsen.

The patient was sent home on the second postoperative day.

One-fourth of the staff was ill with the flu.

Name _____ Date _____

Exercise 8.1 Building Your Medical Vocabulary

Directions Define the following word forms.

Term	Definition
Term	**Definition**
1. a, an	_____
2. cysto	_____
3. dys	_____
4. graph	_____
5. hemato	_____
6. hyper	_____
7. litho	_____
8. nephro	_____
9. nocti	_____
10. oligo	_____
11. -osis	_____
12. -plasia	_____
13. pyo	_____
14. -scopy	_____
15. supra	_____
16. -tripsy	_____
17. -trophy	_____
18. uretero	_____
19. urethro	_____
20. uria	_____

Exercise 8.2 Matching Symptoms and Disease Descriptions

Directions Match the symptom or disease in Column 2 with the definition in Column 1.

Column 1	Column 2
____ 1. pus in urine	a. anuria
____ 2. voiding at night	b. calculus
____ 3. inability to control urination	c. colic
____ 4. inflammation of urethra	d. cystitis
____ 5. urine in bladder after voiding	e. dysuria
____ 6. high blood pressure	f. edema
____ 7. no urine	g. frequency
____ 8. spasms of crampy pain	h. hypertension
____ 9. narrowing of meatus	i. incontinence
____ 10. stone	j. nephrolithiasis
____ 11. excess fluid in tissue	k. nocturia
____ 12. inflammation of ureter	l. pyelonephritis
____ 13. urinating often	m. pyuria
____ 14. the condition of having a kidney stone	n. residual urine
____ 15. painful voiding	o. stenosis
____ 16. inflammation of bladder	p. ureteritis
____ 17. inflammation of kidney	q. urethritis

Exercise 8.3 Working with Abbreviations

Directions Provide the meanings of the following abbreviations.

1. CVA _____

2. IVP _____

3. KUB _____

4. UA _____

5. UC _____

6. UTI _____

Exercise 8.4 Applying Your Editing Skill

Directions Circle the correct answer in each of the following statements.

1. The patient had *necrosis / nephrosis* on his left great toe from lack of treatment to the wound.

2. We will see the patient for urinary *follow up / follow-up / followup* in 2 weeks.

3. The patient was ordered to be on a *healthy / healthful* diet for 7 days before her chemotherapy.

4. Upon palpation, the doctor found the patient's *prostate / prostrate* to be enlarged.

5. On the *fifth / 5th* day of medication, the patient is to cut the dosage in *half / 1/2*.

6. The x-ray and exams found a small *calculus / callus* in the bladder.

7. Next week *1/3 / one-third* of the doctors will attend an out-of-town conference.

8. Her *check up / check-up / checkup* was delayed for 1 month.

9. *Follow up / Follow-up / Followup* with Dr. Larsen next week to review the test results.

10. On the *third / 1/3* Friday of each month, the office will close at noon.

11. The *calculus / callus* on the patient's elbow needed a softening ointment.

12. The patient was *prostate / prostrate* with grief.

HINTS FOR TRANSCRIPTION

Before you begin the transcription for this chapter, be sure you know the following items.

Commonly Dictated Phrases

There was no costovertebral angle (CVA) tenderness.

No flank pain.

There was suprapubic tenderness on palpation.

The specific gravity is 1.020. (*pronounced as ten-twenty*)

There was 2+ edema. (*pronounced as two plus*)

The patient was prepped and draped. (*referring to preparation and draping the area with linens*)

The cath specimen revealed 10–20 rbc's/hpf. (*red blood cells per high-power field*)

Terminology

- Catheters are measured in sizes such as French Number 24, transcribed as #24 French.
- Review the abbreviations for milliequivalent, gram, and milligram.
- The terms *dilation* and *dilatation* are used interchangeably.
- The use of cc (cubic centimeter) is gradually being replaced by milliliter (ml or mL), which is the correct unit for volume.

MEDICAL DOCUMENT TRANSCRIPTION

You are now ready to transcribe the dictation for Chapter 8.

 The dictation for this chapter is by Lee W. Kim, MD. Remember to properly identify each report in the upper right corner.

Chapter 8, Item 1
Your Name
Current Date

---

8 TRANSCRIPTION CHECKOFF SHEET

Use the transcription checkoff sheet to record your work and track your progress as a medical transcriptionist.

DOCTOR DICTATING Lee W. Kim, MD
TYPE OF DICTATION Chart notes, history and physical, and letter
DATE OF TRANSCRIPTION April 17, 20—

Item Number	Patient	Date Started	Date Completed	Grade/ Number of Errors
8.1	Lia Yen			
8.2	Sarah Adair			
8.3	Adella Nash			
8.4	Sharon Tanaka			
8.5	Letter to Barry Reinhart, MD Urology Department, Suite 302 6500 Eagle Street, Denver, CO 80239 RE: Quentin Thorne			
8.6	Betty Nikolai			
8.7	Luisa Enright			
8.8	Eugene Edwards			
8.9	Juan Verdez			
8.10	Carlos Hermanez			
8.11	Mara Kazer			
8.12	Anita Stokes			

The Reproductive System and Obstetrics

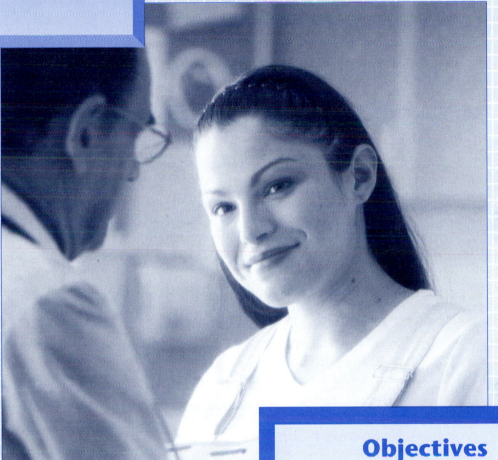

Routine examinations of pregnant patients help ensure the health of the baby and of the mother. *What terms are associated with the patient's medical record over the course of a normal pregnancy?*

Objectives

After completing this chapter, you will be able to

1. Use correct terms when transcribing medical documents covering the functions, assessment, conditions, procedures, and medications of the reproductive system.
2. Transcribe obstetrical chart notes from assigned dictation.
3. Correctly transcribe symbols and numbers from assigned dictation.
4. Apply appropriate AAMT style guidelines to edit and format medical documents.

The anatomical structures of male and female human beings are different. However, both systems consist of sex glands (gonads), passageways, and accessory structures. Hormones from the pituitary gland influence functions of this system. The reproductive system has the following functions: reproduction, production of hormones, and sexual gratification.

Organs of the Male

The male reproductive system is shown in Figure 9.1. The *scrotum* is the sac that contains and maintains the temperature of the two *testes* (testicles), which produce *sperm* and the hormone *testosterone*. Testosterone is essential for development of secondary male characteristics and an increase in skeletal muscle mass. Sperm are stored in the *epididymis* of the testis before entering the *vas deferens*, the muscular tube leading through the *inguinal canal* in the *groin* where the leg meets the body, into the pelvic cavity.

The vas with its accompanying blood vessels and nerves is called the *spermatic cord*. The vas travels through the *prostate gland*, which surrounds the urethra just below the bladder. Fluid is secreted from the prostate and is added to the *semen*, where it aids in the motility of the sperm and in neutralizing the acidity of urine. The vas joins the *urethra*, located within the *penis* (*phallus*). The end (head) of the penis (referred to as *glans penis*) is covered by the *foreskin* (*prepuce*).

The scrotum and penis are the male *external genitalia*. Accessory structures include the *seminal vesicles* and *bulbourethral glands*, which add alkaline fluid to the semen.

Figure 9.1

The Male Reproductive System

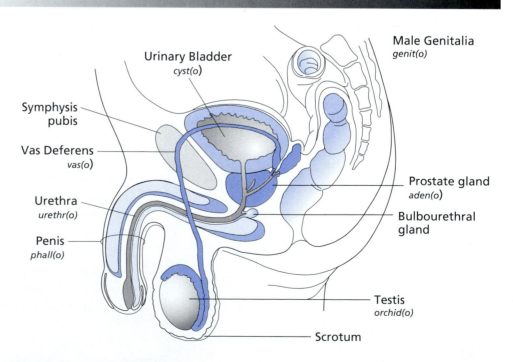

Organs of the Female

The female reproductive system is shown in Figure 9.2. The two *ovaries* are located in the pelvic cavity (pelvis) on either side of the uterus and are anchored to the sides of the uterus by ligaments. The ovaries produce eggs for reproduction and the hormones *estrogen* and *progesterone*. Estrogen is essential for development of female characteristics, including *menstruation*, or *menses*. Progesterone influences the preparation of the endometrial lining of the uterus and the maintenance of a pregnancy.

Several pituitary hormones affect release of the egg from the ovary (*ovulation*), as well as the phases of the menstrual cycle. The *uterine* (*fallopian*) tubes are attached to the right and left sides of the *uterus* near the ovaries. They open into the uterus which is located between the bladder and the rectum. The ovaries and the tubes are referred to as the *adnexa* (adnexum, singular). The *myometrium* is the muscular layer of the uterus, and the *endometrium* is the inner layer that is shed during menses. The lower necklike portion of the uterus is the *cervix*, from which the Papanicolaou (*Pap*) smear is taken.

The *cervical os* opens into the *vagina*, which is lined with mucous membrane arranged in many folds called *rugae*. The upper region of the vagina, surrounding the cervix, is known as the *cul-de-sac*. The muscular vagina extends from the uterus to the *vulva* (*external genitalia*).

External genitalia include the *mons pubis* (the fat pad anterior to the symphysis pubis bone), the *labia minora and majora* (folds of skin and tissue covering the vaginal opening), and the *clitoris* (a small mass of erectile tissue at the apex of the labia). Accessory structures of the female reproductive system include the *Bartholin, Skene's*, and *urethral glands* (abbreviated as *BSU*) and the *hymen*. The *perineum* is the external area between the vulva and the anus in the female.

Figure 9.2

The Female
Reproductive System

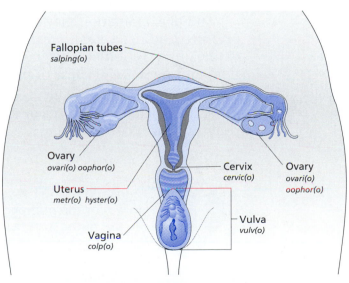

Female genitalia

Mammary Glands

Mammary glands or *breasts* are located anterior to the pectoralis major chest muscle between the second and sixth ribs, lateral to the *sternum* (breast bone), and extend to the *axilla* (armpit). The breasts are composed of *adipose tissue* (fat), lobes of glandular tissues, and the excretory ducts. The *nipples*, at about the fifth rib, contain the openings of the milk ducts. Surrounding the nipples is a circular area of pigmented skin called the *areola*. Breast development begins at puberty in the female and is influenced by hormonal function.

9.2 Clinical Assessment

External genitalia are examined for signs of irritation and/or infection. These include redness, swelling, rash, discharge, and lesions. The prostate is examined digitally through the rectum to determine size, shape, and consistency. Two procedures are performed on the female internal genitalia. In one procedure they are examined with the use of a speculum (instrument). In the other, the bimanual examination, both hands are used; one hand is on the lower abdomen while the examiner's finger pushes internally. This examination is performed to assist in determining changes in or abnormalities of the pelvic organs.

The usual protocol for clinical assessment of a pregnant patient is as follows:

- An appointment for confirmation of the pregnancy

- An initial OB (obstetrics) visit that includes a complete physical exam with Pap smear early in the pregnancy

- Monthly routine OB checks until the eighth month, when routine visits may take place every 2 weeks

- Weekly visits near the end of the term

An OB examination may include the hemoglobin count, blood pressure reading, weight, presence of edema, size of uterus or fundal height, position of fetus, heart rate of fetus (FHT), cervical dilation, and presence of sugar or protein in the urine.

The postpartum checkup is completed about 6 weeks after delivery and includes a Pap smear with, perhaps, recommendations regarding birth control issues.

STYLE TIP

Pregnancy and deliveries are expressed using the words *gravida* for the number of pregnancies and *para* to indicate the number of deliveries.

9.3 Symptoms and Disease Conditions

KEY *terms* The following symptoms and disease conditions apply to the reproductive system. Each term on this list is pronounced at the beginning of the dictation for this chapter. Study the list carefully, practicing pronunciation and building word recognition. Be sure you can spell each term correctly.

TERM	PRONUNCIATION	MEANING
AIDS		acquired immunodeficiency syndrome
atrophic	(ă-trof´ik)	wasting of tissue
cancer	(kan´ser)	malignant growth
cervicitis	(ser-vi-sī´tis)	inflammation of mucosa of the cervix
Chlamydia	(kla-mid´ē-ă)	type of venereal disease
cystic breast disease	(sis´tik)	formation of fluid or semisolid sac of breast tissue
cystocele	(sis´tō-sēl)	herniation of bladder into vaginal wall
dysmenorrhea	(dis-men-ōr-ē´ă)	menstrual cramps
dysplasia	(dis-plā´zē-ă)	abnormal tissue development
endometriosis	(en´dō-mē-trē-ō´sis)	formation of endometrial tissue in the pelvic cavity outside the uterus
epididymitis	(ep-i-did-i-mī´tis)	inflammation of epididymis
erosion	(ē-rō´zhŭn)	wearing away
eversion	(ē-ver´zhŭn)	turning outward
gonorrhea (GC)	(gon-ō-rē´ă)	type of venereal disease
herpes	(her´pēz)	type of venereal disease
human Papilloma virus (HPV)	(pap-i-lō´mă)	type of venereal disease
inguinal hernia	(ing´gwi-năl)	hernia located in the groin
introitus	(in-trō´i-tŭs)	entrance
mastalgia	(mas-tal´jē-ă)	breast pain
menses	(men´sēz)	menstrual period
menopause	(men´ō-pawz)	cessation of menses
menorrhagia	(men-ō-rā´jē-ă)	excessive bleeding at time of period
metrorrhagia	(mē-trō-rā´jē-ă)	bleeding between periods
oligomenorrhea	(ol´i-gō-men-ō-rē´ă)	scanty menstruation
orchitis	(ōr-kī´tis)	inflammation of the testis
osteoporosis	(os´tē-ō-pō-rō´sis)	reduction in bone density
pelvic inflammatory disease (PID)		inflammation of uterus, tubes, and ovaries
premenstrual syndrome (PMS)		group of symptoms occurring before the menstrual period
prolapse of uterus	(prō-laps´)	displacement of uterus into vagina
pruritus		itching
rectocele	(rek´tō-sēl)	herniation of rectum into vaginal wall

TERM	PRONUNCIATION	MEANING
ruga (rugae)	(rū´gă, rū´gē)	fold, ridge
sexually transmitted diseases (STDs)		venereal diseases
Trichomonas	(trik-ō-mō´nas)	parasitic infection
vaginosis	(vaj-i-nō´sis)	bacterial infection of vagina
wrinkle	(ring´kl)	fold, crease

9.4 Laboratory Procedures

KEY*terms* Tests that are used in the dictation for this chapter are listed below.

Pregnancy may be confirmed by blood or urine tests.

Blood is tested to confirm human immunodeficiency virus (HIV).

The following infections may be identified by a technique called wet prep/mount from penile and vaginal secretions:

TERM	PRONUNCIATION
Chlamydia	(kla-mid´ē-ă)
Gonococcus (GC)	(gon-ō-kok´ŭs)
herpesvirus	(her´pēz-vǐ´rŭs)
Trichomonas and yeast (T&Y)	(trik-o-mō´nas)

9.5 Radiology Procedures

KEY*terms* The radiology terms that appear in the dictation for this chapter are described below. Study each term's spelling, pronunciation, and meaning so you are prepared for transcription.

TERM	PRONUNCIATION	MEANING
bone density		status of bone, useful in determining risk of osteoporosis
mammogram	(mam´ō-gram)	breast x-ray
ultrasound	(ŭl´tră-sownd)	detects liquid or solid masses such as cysts and tumors and determines gestational size

9.6 Medical and Surgical Procedures

KEY*terms* The procedural terms that appear in the dictation for this chapter are described below. Study each term's spelling, pronunciation, and meaning so you are prepared for transcription.

TERM	PRONUNCIATION	MEANING
breast self-exam		examination of one's own breast tissue for abnormal lumps
cesarean section (C-section)	(se-zā´rē-ăn)	abdominal incision for removal of fetus
circumcision	(ser-kŭm-sizh´ŭn)	removal of penile foreskin
cryotherapy	(krī-ō-thăr´ă-pē)	use of cold for treatment
cystorrhaphy	(sis-tōr´ă-fē)	suturing of urinary bladder
dilatation & curettage (D&C)	(dil-ă-tā´shŭn and kyū-rĕ-tahzh´)	stretching and scraping uterine cavity
hysterectomy	(his-ter-ek´tō-mē)	removal of uterus
laparoscopy	(lap-ă-ros´kō-pē)	viewing internal abdominal organs with endoscope
lumpectomy	(lŭm-pek´tō-mē)	removal of lump from breast
mastectomy	(mas-tek´tō-mē)	excision of breast
oophorosalpingectomy	(ō-of´ōr-ō-sal-pin-jek´tō-mē)	removal of ovary and tube
Pap smear		test for cervical cancer
Sitz bath	(sitz)	sitting and soaking area from tailbone to lower abdomen in a tub of warm water
testicular self-exam		examination of one's own scrotum for abnormal lumps
uterine suspension	(yū´ter-in)	tightening structures that hold uterus in place
vasectomy	(va-sek´tō-mē)	removal of segment of vas deferens

9.7 Medications

KEY*terms* The medications that appear in the dictation for this chapter are described below. Study each medication's spelling, pronunciation, and classification.

TERM	PRONUNCIATION	CLASSIFICATION
doxycycline	(dok-sē-sī´klēn)	antibiotic
Estraderm	(es´tra-derm)	hormone
Motrin	(mō´trin)	NSAID, analgesic, antipyretic
tamoxifen	(tă-mok´si-fen)	antineoplastic

9.8 Related Terms

KEY_terms_ The following terms appear in the dictation for this chapter. Study the spelling, pronunciation, and meaning of these terms.

TERM	PRONUNCIATION	MEANING
axillary	(ak´sil-ār-ē)	pertaining to the armpit
basic metabolic panel	(met-ă-bol´ik)	group of routine blood tests that determine the general state of health
clubbing	(klŭb´ing)	abnormality of fingertips indicative of chronic lung disease
cyanosis	(sī-ă-nō´sis)	bluish tinge to skin due to circulatory or respiratory problems
cytobrush	(sī-tō´brŭsh)	used to collect Pap smear specimen
incarceration	(in-kar´ser-ă-shŭn)	being trapped
Jackson-Pratt drain	(jak´son prat)	tube used for wound drainage
pendulous	(pen´dū-lŭs)	hanging freely
strangulation	(strang´gyū-lā´shŭn)	constriction of blood flow
vertigo	(ver´ti-gō)	dizziness

9.9 OB Terms

KEY_terms_ The following terms are related to obstetrics. Study the spelling, pronunciation, and meaning of these terms.

TERM	PRONUNCIATION	MEANING
breech	(brēch)	buttocks presenting at vaginal opening at time of delivery
cephalopelvic disproportion	(sef´ă-lō-pel´vik)	size of fetal head to maternal pelvis
eclampsia	(ek-lamp´sē-ă)	toxic condition of pregnancy with hypertension, proteinuria, edema, and/or convulsions
ectopic	(ek-top´ik)	misplaced
episiotomy	(e-piz-ē-ot´ō-mē)	incision of vulva to facilitate delivery of fetus
fetal heart tones (FHT)		pulse rate of fetus
fundus	(fŭn´dŭs)	upper rounded part of uterus
gestation	(jes-tā´shŭn)	pregnancy
gravid	(grav´id)	pregnant
gravida	(grav´id-ă)	pregnant woman
parous	(par´ŭs)	having given birth
partum	(par´tŭm)	delivery of fetus
vertex	(ver´teks)	top of the skull

9.10   Build Your Editing Skills

KEY_terms_ In this section, you will gain the skills you need to correctly transcribe medical documents.

Selecting the Right Word

The words listed here are often confused in transcription because they sound alike when dictated but have different meanings. Study the words carefully so you will be able to select the correct term according to the context of the dictation.

TERM	MEANING	EXAMPLE
fatal	pertaining to death	The patient was diagnosed with a fatal disease.
fecal	pertaining to matter discharged during a bowel movement	Fecal matter was found in the lower cecum.
fetal	relating to the unborn	The fetal heart tones decelerated during labor.
inter (prefix)	between, among	The psychologist told the patient to practice interpersonal situations before the next session.
intra (prefix)	within, during	The intrauterine exam revealed a small fibrous tumor.
perineal	relating to the space between the anus and genital organs	Before delivery, the perineal area was thoroughly cleansed.
peroneal	relating to the fibula, lateral side of the leg	An incision was made along the peroneal nerve to proceed with vein stripping.

Using the Correct Style

Medical transcriptionists use correct style when preparing medical documents.

Study the following obstetrical guidelines. (The basic medical transcription guidelines are in Appendix A.)

GUIDELINE

Use *C-section* if dictated; otherwise, do not abbreviate *cesarean section*.

EXAMPLE

The patient's cesarean section was scheduled for 2 p.m.

STYLE TIP

Do not capitalize *cesarean,* but capitalize the *C* and use a hyphen in *C-section.*

Use Arabic numbers with GPA terminology: *gravida* (number of pregnancies), *para* (number of births), and *abortus* (abortions). Separate each with commas. If one of the numbers is zero (0), then the terms are spelled out.

Obstetric history was gravida 3, para 2, abortus 1.
OBSTETRIC HISTORY: G3, P2, A1.
OBSTETRIC HISTORY: gravida 2, para 2, abortus 0.

Obstetric history may be described using TPAL terminology: *T* (term infants), *P* (premature infants), *A* (abortions), and *L* (living children). Use Arabic numbers and separate with hyphens if abbreviated.

OBSTETRIC HISTORY: 2 term infants, 1 premature infant, 0 abortions, 2 living children.
OBSTETRIC HISTORY: 2-1-0-2.

Also, some physicians use a combination of GPA and TPAL terminology.

The patient was gravida 2, para 2-0-0-2.

The terms *genitalia* and *menses* are always plural.

The genitalia were normal in appearance.
Menses began at age 12.

Name _____   Date _____

Exercise 9.1   Building Your Medical Vocabulary

Directions Define the following word forms.

TERM	DEFINITION
1. adeno	_____
2. -algia	_____
3. ante	_____
4. -cele	_____
5. cervico	_____
6. colpo	_____
7. dys	_____
8. endo	_____
9. gyneco	_____
10. hystero	_____
11. masto/mammo	_____
12. meno	_____
13. metro	_____
14. oophoro	_____
15. orchido	_____
16. -rrhagia	_____
17. -rrhea	_____
18. salpingo	_____
19. -tropho	_____
20. vas	_____

Exercise 9.2 Matching Symptoms with Diseases/Procedures

Directions Match the symptom, disease, or procedure in Column 2 with the definition in Column 1.

Column 1

____ 1. abnormal tissue development

____ 2. inflammation of the cervical mucosa

____ 3. excessive breast formation in male

____ 4. menstrual cramps

____ 5. pain in breast

____ 6. bleeding between menstruation cycles

____ 7. itching

____ 8. cessation of menses

____ 9. excessive bleeding during menses

____ 10. inflammation of the testis

____ 11. herniation of rectum into vaginal wall

____ 12. removal of foreskin of penis

____ 13. use of cold treatment

____ 14. scraping within the cervix

____ 15. examination of vagina and cervix with an endoscope

____ 16. excision of breast

____ 17. removal of ovary and tube

Column 2

a. cervicitis

b. circumcision

c. colposcopy

d. cryotherapy

e. dysmenorrhea

f. dysplasia

g. endocervical curettage

h. gynecomastia

i. mastalgia

j. mastectomy

k. menopause

l. menorrhagia

m. metrorrhagia

n. oophorosalpingectomy

o. orchitis

p. pruritus

q. rectocele

Exercise 9.3 Working with Abbreviations

Directions Provide the meanings of the following abbreviations.

1. AIDS   _____

2. BSU   _____

3. C-section _____

4. FHT   _____

5. GC   _____

6. HIV   _____

7. HPV   _____

8. PID   _____

9. PMS   _____

10. STD   _____

Exercise 9.4 Applying Your Editing Skills

Directions Circle the correct term in the following statements.

1. Blood loss *intraoperatively / interoperatively* was 50 cc.

2. The *perineal / peroneal* area was prepped for hemorrhoid surgery.

3. *Fecal / Fatal / Fetal* presentation was at a -3 station.

4. The patient was evaluated for *intermenstrual / intramenstrual* spotting.

5. The patient was *gravida 4, P2, A2 / G4, P2, A2.*

6. Her first child was delivered by *c-section / Cesarean Section / C-section.*

7. An *interuterine / intrauterine* biopsy will be obtained under local anesthesia.

8. The 23-year-old female was *gravida 3, para 3, abortus 0 / G3-P3-A0.*

9. The patient was depressed because of her mother's *fatal / fetal / fecal* condition.

10. The patient is undergoing psychological therapy to evaluate her *intersexual / intrasexual* skills.

11. Rectal exam showed the stitches to be healing in the *perineal / peroneal* area.

12. *Fatal / Fecal / Fetal* heart tones could not be heard.

13. OBSTETRIC HISTORY: *3-0-1-2 / 3, 0, 1, 2.*

14. The young patient needed *interpartum / intrapartum* assistance to help with breathing techniques before delivering the twins.

15. The resident surgeon performed the *Cesarean / cesarean* section.

HINTS FOR TRANSCRIPTION

Before you begin the transcription for this chapter, be sure you know the following items.

Commonly Dictated Phrases

Left adnexa are not palpable.

Breasts are symmetric.

There is no discrete nipple discharge or adenopathy.

Breasts have no masses, discharge, or tenderness.

There is no nipple dimpling, discharge, or mass.

The prostate is smooth and nontender.

The prostate is 2+ and boggy.

There was no costovertebral angle (CVA) tenderness.

Fundal height, 30 cm; vertex presenting, high and floating; FHTs, 150.

Pap smear was negative.

MEDICAL DOCUMENT TRANSCRIPTION

You are now ready to transcribe the dictation for Chapter 9.

The dictation for this chapter is by Debra Litman, MD. Remember to properly identify each report in the upper right corner, as shown here:

Chapter 9, Item 1
Your Name
Current Date

9 TRANSCRIPTION CHECKOFF SHEET

Use the transcription checkoff sheet to record your work and track your progress as a medical transcriptionist.

DOCTOR DICTATING Debra Litman, MD
TYPE OF DICTATION Chart notes, history and physical, and letters
DATE OF TRANSCRIPTION April 19, 20—

Item Number	Patient	Date Started	Date Completed	Grade/ Number of Errors
9.1	Richard Kaplan			
9.2	Letter to Belinda Hegdahl, MD, RE: Jared Hoffmeier			
9.3	Suzette Meyers			
9.4	Letter to Donna Hooley			
9.5	Paula Geiger			
9.6	Soon Lee Yim			
9.7	Shelley Ellis			
9.8	Chi Hyatt			
9.9	Letter to Mia Young, MD, RE: Ann Sankaaran			
9.10	Letter to Belinda Hegdahl, MD, RE: Leah Ahmann			
9.11	Sandra Pascoe			
9.12	Tasha Sprague			

TRANSCRIPTION TEST 3

After the Chapter 9 transcription has been corrected and returned to you for review, you are ready to take the third transcription test. Obtain the test recording from your instructor.

CHAPTER 10

The Musculoskeletal System

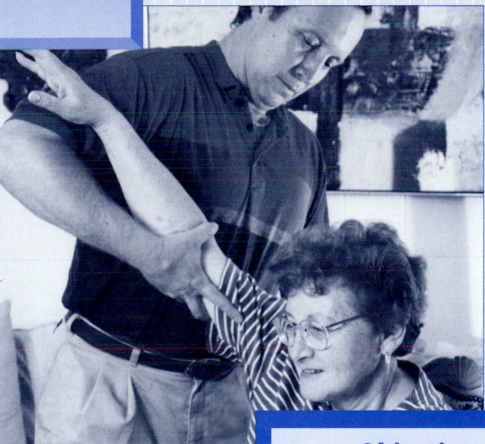

Restoring normal movement is the goal of many procedures relating to the musculoskeletal systems. *What are some of the terms used to describe conditions of the bones and muscles?*

Objectives

After completing this chapter, you will be able to

1. Use correct terms when transcribing medical documents covering musculoskeletal system functions, assessment, conditions, procedures, and medications.
2. Use reference material as needed for the correct spelling of nouns and adjectives.
3. Locate the major bones and muscles of the body using diagrams.
4. Apply appropriate AAMT style guidelines to edit and format medical documents.

10.1 Understanding the Musculoskeletal System

The musculoskeletal system includes the bones and muscles with their attached ligaments and tendons. Their functioning is interrelated with the endocrine system, which produces hormones that affect growth, and with the nervous system, which sends impulses that affect their movement. An adequate blood supply is essential to the functioning of muscles and bones.

10.2 Bones

The bones have the following functions:

- **Framework** The muscles are attached to the bones to provide the framework of the body.

- **Protection** The bones provide protection of the internal organs.

- **Movement** The muscles provide movement of the body.

- **Storage of calcium** Bones, teeth, nerves, and other structures need calcium in order to function properly.

- **Production of blood cells** Red and white blood cells are formed in the bone marrow.

Bones are covered with a tough membrane called the *periosteum*. The ends of the bones are covered with *cartilage*.

The connection of two or more bones is called a *joint* or an *articulation*. Some joints, especially those that move a lot, contain a sac filled with *synovial fluid*, which allows for ease in movement. A bursa is a fluid-filled sac found in areas that are subject to friction (that is, where a tendon passes over a bone). Joints may be identified by using the names of the connecting bones and/or their location, such as temporomandibular joint, sacroiliac joint, costochondral junction, proximal interphalangeal joint (PIP), or metacarpophalangeal joint (MCP), and so forth.

Joints also have a tough band of tissue, a *ligament*, that connects bone to bone and reinforces the joint. A common group of ligaments are the collaterals in the knee.

Tendons attach bones to muscles. An example is the Achilles tendon in the heel region.

10.3 Bones: Anatomical Landmarks

KEY_terms_ Bones have many landmarks, the most important of which are identified on the next page.

TERM	PRONUNCIATION	MEANING
acromion	(ă-krō´mē-on)	bony projection forming part of shoulder joint
condyle	(kon´dĭl)	bulge (on a bone)
epiphysis	(e-pif´i-sis)	end, or growing region, of a long bone
fontanel	(fon´tă-nel´)	"soft spot" or joint in skull (cranium) of infants before bones have fused
head		upper portion of the arm and leg bones
lamina	(lam´i-nă)	a region of vertebra
malleolus (plural—malleoli)	(ma-lē´ō-lŭs) (ma-lē´ō-lĭ)	projection on either side of lower leg (the ankle)
sciatic notch	(sī-at´ik)	depression in ischial bone
shaft	(shaft)	midportion of a long bone
sinus	(sī´nŭs)	air pocket in bone to make bone lighter
styloid	(stī´loyd)	sharp projection
trochanter	(trō-kan´ter)	big bulge on the upper leg bone
tuberosity	(tū´ber-os´i-tē)	big bulge or knob

10.4 Locating the Major Bones

Using standard references, enter the appropriate number from Figure 10.1 next to the bone shown on page 148.

_____	calcaneus	(kal-kā´nē-ŭs)
_____	carpals	(kar´păls)
_____	cervical vertebra	(ser´vi-kăl ver´tĕ-bră)
_____	clavicle	(klav´i-kl)
_____	coccyx	(kok´siks)
_____	cranium	(krā´nē-ŭm)
_____	femur	(fē´mŭr)
_____	fibula	(fib´yū-lă)
_____	humerus	(hyū´mer-ŭs)
_____	ilium	(il´ē-ŭm)
_____	lumbar vertebra	(lŭm´bar ver´tĕ-bră)
_____	metacarpals	(met´ă-kar´păls)
_____	metatarsals	(met´ă-tar´săls)
_____	patella	(pa-tel´ă)
_____	phalanges	(fā-lan´jēz)
_____	radius	(rā´dē-ŭs)
_____	ribs	(ribs)
_____	sacrum	(sā´krŭm)
_____	scapula	(skap´yū-lă)
_____	sternum	(ster´num)
_____	tarsals	(tar´săls)

_____ thoracic vertebra   (thō-ras´ik ver´tĕ-bră)

_____ tibia   (tib´ē-ă)

_____ ulna   (ŭl´nă)

Figure 10.1

Major Bones
of the Body

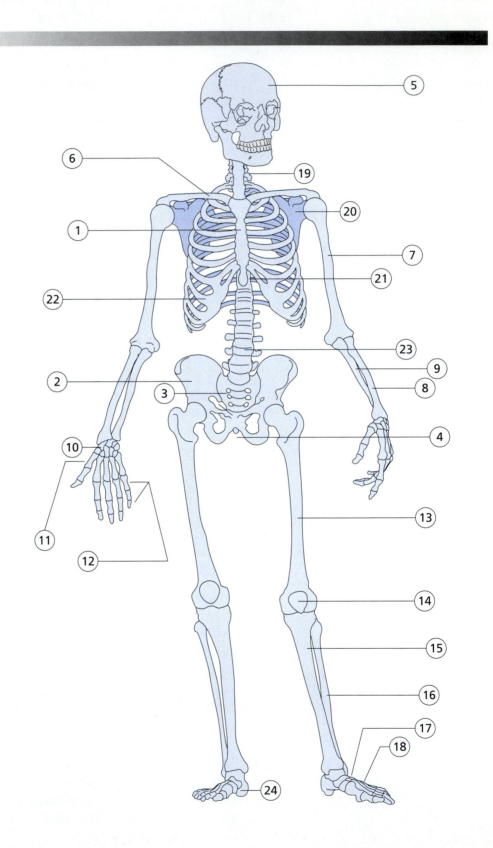

10.5 | Muscles

Muscles attach to bones of the skeleton, and they make up the walls of internal organs including the heart. The nervous system is involved with stimulation of the muscles to initiate muscle function. There are more than 600 muscles in the body. This chapter concentrates on the skeletal muscles.

Muscles have the following functions:

- **Movement** This includes movement of the bones as well as activity of the internal organs.

- **Maintenance of posture** This involves controlling muscles to keep the body in normal functioning positions.

- **Heat production** This entails producing body heat from the movement of the skeletal muscles.

Bones and muscles work together to produce movement of body parts. They frequently work in pairs. Refer to Figure 2.1 in Chapter 2 to review six common joint movements.

10.6 | Locating the Major Muscles

Using standard references, enter the appropriate numbers from Figure 10.2 on page 150, next to the common muscles shown below:

_____ abdominal
_____ anterior thigh
_____ anterior lower leg
_____ between shoulder blades
_____ buttocks
_____ calf
_____ chest
_____ inner upper arm
_____ lower back
_____ major neck muscle
_____ outer upper arm
_____ posterior thigh
_____ shoulder cap
_____ upper back, shoulder-to-shoulder and across vertebrae

Figure 10.2

Major Muscles of
the Body

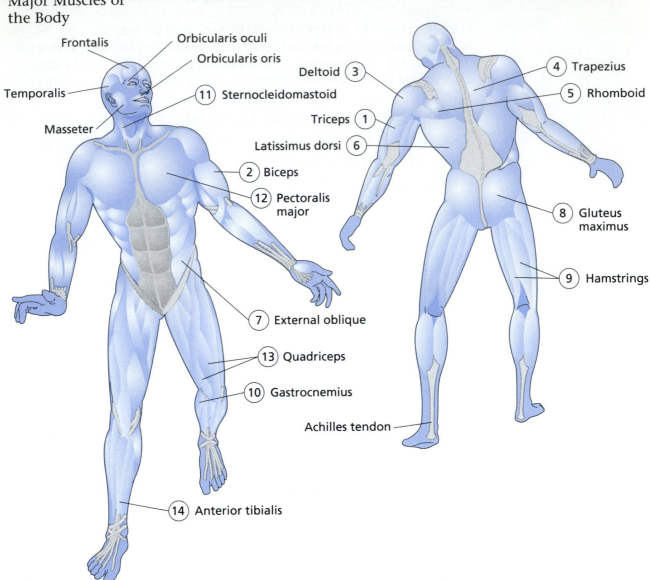

Frontalis

Orbicularis oculi

Orbicularis oris

Temporalis

Masseter

⑪ Sternocleidomastoid

Deltoid ③

Triceps ①

Latissimus dorsi ⑥

② Biceps

⑫ Pectoralis
major

④ Trapezius

⑤ Rhomboid

⑧ Gluteus
maximus

⑨ Hamstrings

⑦ External oblique

⑬ Quadriceps

⑩ Gastrocnemius

Achilles tendon

⑭ Anterior tibialis

10.7   Clinical Assessment

The examiner observes this system for muscle functioning: complete range of motion (ROM) of joints, muscle strength, bulk, and
tone, as well as for pain, stiffness, and limitation of movements.

STYLE TIP

Muscle strength is graded on a scale of 0 to 5 (contrac-
tion against resistance); 0 indicates complete paralysis; 5
indicates normal strength, also referred to as intact.

Dictated: Muscle strength is five over five in the right
hand and two over five in the left hand.

Transcribed: Muscle strength is 5/5 in the right hand
and 2/5 in the left hand.

The nervous system works with the musculoskeletal system; thus associated functions are tested. These include deep tendon reflex testing (DTRs) of knee, ankle, patella, triceps, and biceps. Radial and ulnar jerks are also evaluated.

Circulation is observed, since it is often compromised during injury when there is swelling and/or broken blood vessels.

10.8   Maneuvers, Signs, or Tests

Following is a list of maneuvers, signs, or tests that apply to the examination of the musculoskeletal system. Review a reference source for explanations.

Apley grind
apprehension sign
deep tendon reflexes (DTRs)
drawer sign
heel-and-toe walk
impingement sign
McMurray test
Patrick's test

Phalen test
range of motion (ROM)
  active
  passive
spring test
straight-leg raise test
Tinel's sign

STYLE TIP

Note that some references show possession with 's; others do not use the 's. The AAMT recommends that the possessive form not be used with eponymic terms.

10.9   Symptoms and Disease Conditions

 The following symptoms and disease conditions apply to the musculoskeletal system. Each term on this list is pronounced at the beginning of the dictation for this chapter. Study the list carefully, practicing pronunciation and building word recognition. Be sure you can spell each term correctly.

TERM	PRONUNCIATION	MEANING
alignment	(ă-līn´ment)	proper position
arthritis	(ar-thrī´tis)	joint inflammation
degenerative		deterioration of joint structures
gouty	(gow´tē)	deposits of crystals in joints
rheumatoid	(rū´mă-toyd)	also constitutional symptoms
avulsion	(ă-vŭl´shŭn)	separation
bursitis	(ber-sī´tus)	inflammation of bursa
carpal tunnel syndrome	(kar´păl)	symptoms such as pain and weakness in the wrist caused by pressure on median nerve
Colles fracture	(kōl´ez)	fractured radius with displacement

TERM	PRONUNCIATION	MEANING
costochondritis	(kos´tō-kon-drī´tis)	inflammation of cartilage between ribs
crepitus	(krep´i-tŭs)	crackling or bubbling sound or feeling
degenerative disk disease (DDD)	(dē-jen´er-ă-tiv)	deterioration of disk
degenerative joint disease (DJD)		deterioration of joints
dislocation	(dis´lō-kā´shŭn)	displacement; disruption of proper position
effusion	(e-fū´zhŭn)	excessive fluid in joint space
fracture	(frak´chūr)	break
herniated disk	(her´nē-ā-ted)	disk that protrudes
impingement	(im-pinj´ment)	beyond the usual limit or location
myositis	(mī-ō-sī´tis)	inflammation of muscle
nonunion	(non´yūn-yŭn)	unhealed fracture site
radiculopathy	(ra-dik´yū-lop´ă-thē)	disease of spinal nerve roots
sprain	(sprān)	twisting-type injury
strain	(strān)	muscle injury caused by overuse or improper use
tendonitis or tendinitis	(ten-dō-nī´tis or ten-di-nī´tis)	inflammation of tendon
whiplash	(hwip´lash)	neck injury when struck from behind

10.10 Laboratory Tests

KEYterms Laboratory studies are performed for the diagnosis of many conditions. A test that is used in the dictation for this chapter is listed below. Refer to Appendix D for a detailed explanation.

TERM	PRONUNCIATION	MEANING
uric acid	(ur´ik)	byproduct of metabolism causing crystal or stone formation resulting in gout or kidney stones

10.11 Radiology Procedures

KEYterms The radiology terms that appear in the dictation for this chapter are described on the next page. Study each term's spelling, pronunciation, and meaning so you are prepared for transcription.

TERM	MEANING
C-spine	x-ray of cervical spine
MRI (magnetic resonance imaging)	used to diagnose knee ligament injuries, shoulder injuries, and disk problems
plain films	taken to outline bones, looking for abnormalities; x-rays that do not use contrast media

10.12 Medical and Surgical Procedures

KEY *terms* The procedural terms that appear in the dictation for this chapter are described below. Study each term's spelling, pronunciation, and meaning so you are prepared for transcription.

TERM	PRONUNCIATION	MEANING
arthroscopy	(ar-thros´kŏ-pē)	visualization of a joint using special surgical instrument
cast	(kast)	application of rigid material to prevent movement
crutch	(krŭtch)	device used for support (usually under the armpit) when walking
electromyogram (EMG)	(ē-lek-trō-mī´ō-gram)	a graphic representation of muscle function that uses electrical stimulation
immobilization	(i-mō´bi-li-ză-shŭn)	prevention of movement
joint replacement (prosthesis)	(pros´thē-sis)	to replace degenerative joint or repair a fracture
laminectomy	(lam´i-nek´tō-mē)	removal of part of a vertebra
physical therapy		use of water, electricity, massage, exercise, etc., to evaluate and treat disabilities
reduction	(rē-dŭk´shŭn)	realigning a fracture
closed		manipulation and immobilization without surgical incision
internal fixation		immobilization with screws, nails, plates, or rods
open		incision needed to perform realignment
sling	(sling)	piece of cloth looped under arm and around shoulder and/or neck for arm support
splint	(splint)	temporary device to prevent movement of a bone

10.13   Medications

KEY *terms*   The medications that appear in the dictation for this chapter are described below. Study each medication's spelling, pronunciation, and classification.

TERM	PRONUNCIATION	CLASSIFICATION
Aleve	(ă-lēv)	NSAID, analgesic
allopurinol	(al-ō-pyū´ri-nol)	antigout
Aristospan	(ă-rist´ō-span)	cortisone
(triamcinolone)	(trī-am-sin´ō-lōn)	
aspirin	(as´pi-rin)	analgesic, antipyretic
Daypro	(da´prō)	NSAID
Naprosyn	(nap´rō-sin)	analgesic, antipyretic

10.14   Related Terms

KEY *terms*   The following terms appear in the dictation for this chapter. Study the spelling, pronunciation, and meaning of these terms.

TERM	PRONUNCIATION	MEANING
chiropractic	(kī-rō-prak´tik)	method of treating disease by manipulation of the joints
gait	(gāt)	method of walking
laxity	(lak´să-tē)	looseness
neurosensory	(nūr´ō-sen´sŏ-rē)	relating to nerve sensation
neurovascular	(nūr-ō-vas´kyū-lăr)	having to do with nerve blood vessels
numbness	(nŭm´nes)	without feeling
oblique	(ob-lēk´)	slanted position
orthopedics	(ōr-thō-pē´diks)	branch of medicine dealing with conditions of the musculoskeletal system
pivot	(piv´ŏt)	point at which something turns or hinges

10.15 Build Your Editing Skills

In this section, you will gain the skills you need to correctly transcribe medical documents.

Selecting the Right Word

The words listed here are often confused in transcription because they sound alike when dictated but have different meanings. Study the words carefully so you will be able to select the correct term according to the context of the dictation.

TERM/ PRONUNCIATION	MEANING	EXAMPLE
addiction (ă-dĭk´shŭn)	psychological and physiological dependence on a substance	Jan is being admitted to a drug treatment center for her addiction to pain pills.
adduction (ă-dŭk´shŭn)	body part movement toward the middle	The patient's upper strength adduction was within normal limits.
arthrosclerosis (ar´thrō-skler-ō´sis)	stiffness of the joints	Her arthrosclerosis was causing painful extremity movement.
arteriosclerosis and atherosclerosis (ar-tēr´ē-ō-skler-ō´sis) (ath´er-ō-skler-ō´sis)	hardening of the arteries and/or lipid deposits	The patient's elevated blood pressure was caused by arteriosclerosis.
ileum (il´ē-ŭm)	third portion of small intestine	The patient was diagnosed with terminal ileitis, ulcerations, and granulomas occurring in the ileum.
ilium (il´ē-ŭm)	iliac or flank bone; flaring portion of the hip bone	The x-ray of the hip revealed a fracture of the ilium.

Using the Correct Style

Medical transcriptionists use correct style when preparing medical documents. Study the guidelines here to learn the rules for the dictation in this chapter. (The basic medical transcription guidelines are in Appendix A.)

GUIDELINE	EXAMPLE
Use a capital *C, L, T,* or *S* to indicate the vertebral regions (cervical, lumbar, thoracic, or sacral) followed by an Arabic number. Do not use a hyphen between the letter and number or subscript the number; however, a hyphen is used to indicate the space between two vertebrae.	There is mild T1 joint tenderness. The L5-S1 interspace was within normal limits.
Write out nonspecific numerical expressions.	The patient's spouse stated that her husband gave hundreds of reasons why he was not following the physician's advice.
Set off independent clauses that already contain one or more commas and have a conjunction.	If Dr. Larson can see the patient, make an appointment for next week; or if Dr. Wilson has to see the patient, make the appointment as soon as possible.
Compound nouns ending in *on* and *in* are generally hyphenated.	Check-in at the hospital is before 3 p.m. The assistant's run-in with the patient was heard by the entire staff.
Compound nouns ending in *out, over,* and *back* are generally written as one solid word.	There was a breakout of Strep at the school. The feedback from the survey is expected by the end of the week. The new owner's takeover went smoothly.

Name _____ Date _____

Exercise 10.1 Building Your Medical Vocabulary

Directions Match the word form or suffix in Column 2 with its definition in Column 1.

Column 1	Column 2
____ 1. bone	a. arthro
____ 2. straight	b. chiro
____ 3. cartilage	c. chondro
____ 4. joint	d. costo
____ 5. muscle	e. cranio
____ 6. rib	f. myo
____ 7. spinal column	g. ortho
____ 8. skull	h. osteo
____ 9. hand	i. thoraco
____ 10. chest	j. vertebro

Name _____ Date _____

Exercise 10.2 Identifying Bones

Directions Match the following bone or bones in Column 2 with its location in Column 1.

Column 1	Column 2
____ 1. ankle	a. calcaneus
____ 2. forearm, thumb side	b. carpals
____ 3. kneecap	c. cervical region
____ 4. hand	d. clavicle
____ 5. fingers and toes	e. coccyx
____ 6. rib cage	f. cranium
____ 7. lower leg	g. femur
____ 8. vertebral column between ilia	h. humerus
____ 9. skull	i. ilium
____ 10. neck area	j. lumbar region
____ 11. tailbone	k. metacarpals
____ 12. collarbone	l. patella
____ 13. heel	m. phalanges
____ 14. forearm, little-finger side	n. radius
____ 15. thigh	o. sacrum
____ 16. wrist	p. sternum
____ 17. upper arm	q. tarsals
____ 18. hip	r. thorax
____ 19. small of the back	s. tibia
____ 20. breastbone	t. ulna

Exercise 10.3 Matching Symptoms and Conditions

Directions Match the term in Column 2 with its meaning in Column 1.

Column 1	Column 2
____ 1. broken bone	a. alignment
____ 2. inflammation of tendon	b. arthritis
____ 3. inflammation of joint	c. avulsion
____ 4. grating or crackle sound	d. crepitus
____ 5. "pulled" muscle	e. degeneration
____ 6. tissue separation	f. dislocation
____ 7. deterioration of a joint	g. fracture
____ 8. protruding disk	h. herniated
____ 9. in correct position	i. sprain
____ 10. displaced	j. tendinitis

Exercise 10.4 Applying Your Editing Skills

Directions Circle the correct term in the following statements.

1. There was a mild disk bulge between *L2-L3 / L-2 - L-3*.

2. The *turn-over / turnover* of staff has decreased in the past six months.

3. There are *hundreds / 100s* of reasons why I cannot attend the conference.

4. You must change your password *log-in / login* after 50 entries into the computer system.

5. The patient claimed to have an *addiction / adduction* to caffeine.

6. There have been minor changes in the *C-1 / C1* interspace since the last x-ray.

7. The elderly patient showed signs of *arteriosclerosis / arthrosclerosis* in both elbows.

8. The patient was told to stand with both arms at his side before starting *addiction / adduction* exercises.

9. Today's *weigh-in / weighin* for our dieting group will be in Conference Room A.

10. A barium study confirmed a stricture of the *ileum / ilium*.

11. There was a 3-hour *black-out / blackout* in our facility last Saturday.

12. The *print-out / printout* of next week's schedule is on Danny's desk.

13. The interactive counseling session for drug *addiction / adduction* is this afternoon.

14. A bone scan revealed metastases to the femur, vertebra, and *ileum / ilium*.

15. One of the patient's heart problems included *arthrosclerosis / atherosclerosis*.

HINTS FOR TRANSCRIPTION

Before you begin the transcription for this chapter, be sure you know the following items.

Reflexes

Reflexes are graded on a scale of 1 to 4.

> **Dictated** Deep tendon reflexes are two plus over four and symmetric.
>
> **Transcribed** Deep tendon reflexes are 2+/4 and symmetric.

Plurals

Form the plural of words that end in *itis* by dropping the *s* and adding *des*.

> **Singular** arthritis
> **Plural** arthritides

Form the plural of some words ending in *a* by adding an *e*.
Note: Pronunciation of the plural form may be i, ē, or a.

> **Singular** bursa, vertebra
> **Plural** bursae, vertebrae

Form the plural of words that end in *us* by changing the *us* to *i*.

> **Singular** meniscus
> **Plural** menisci

Form the plural of words that end in *nx* by changing the *x* to *g* and add *es*.

> **Singular** phalanx
> **Plural** phalanges

Note that some words, such as biceps, triceps, or quadriceps can be singular or plural.

Commonly Dictated Phrases

> heel-and-toe walking, position sense, light touch, pinprick sensation, and downgoing toes
>
> checking the peripheral pulses, which include radial, ulnar, popliteal, posterior tibial, and dorsalis pedis

---

MEDICAL DOCUMENT TRANSCRIPTION

You are now ready to transcribe the dictation for Chapter 10.

The dictation for this chapter is by John Blackburn, MD. Remember to properly identify each report in the upper right corner.

> Chapter 10, Item 1
> Your Name
> Current Date

---

10 TRANSCRIPTION CHECKOFF SHEET

Use the transcription checkoff sheet to record your work and track your progress as a medical transcriptionist.

DOCTOR DICTATING John Blackburn, MD
TYPE OF DICTATION Chart notes, letters, x-ray reports, and procedure note
DATE OF TRANSCRIPTION April 22, 20—

Item Number	Patient	Date Started	Date Completed	Grade/ Number of Errors
10.1	Joellen Ulrich			
10.2	Joseph Iverson			
10.3	Letter to Arthur Braun, MD, RE: Tom Quam			
10.4	Ben Sankaaran			
10.5	Deann O'Connell			
10.6	Stephan Taggert			
10.7	Tianne St. John			
10.8	Letter to Arthur Braun, MD, RE: Destiny Gomez			
10.9	Rudolph Zakowski			
10.10	Roger Gates			
10.11	Luke Nguyen			
10.12	Rachelle Bacella			
10.13	Lawrence Minick			
10.14	Dana DeMarcos			

CHAPTER

11

The Nervous System

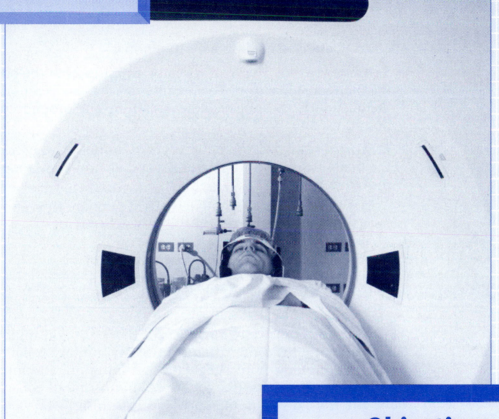

Computed tomography (CT) scans are x-rays that are used to build a computerized cross-sectional illustration of the brain and spinal cord. CT scans help assess the causes of neurological problems. *What other procedures may be used to evaluate neurological conditions?*

Objectives

After completing this chapter, you will be able to

1. Use correct terms when transcribing medical documents covering nervous system functions, assessment, conditions, procedures, and medications.
2. Briefly discuss the correlation between the central and peripheral nervous systems.
3. Apply appropriate AAMT style guidelines to edit and format medical documents.

11.1 Understanding the Nervous System

The nervous system controls and coordinates the body's movements and functions. It also receives sensory input from various parts of the body. This is accomplished by nerves' responding to stimuli. The nervous system consists of nerves, brain, spinal cord, and sense organs.

A nerve is made up of special cells (*neurons*) and their supporting structures. These structures act like a telephone communication or relay system, carrying impulses to and from the body parts and the brain.

Nerves are classified by their functions:

- **Sensory nerves** These nerves carry impulses from the body to the brain or spinal cord. The impulses are known as sensations and include touch, pressure, pain, temperature, and proprioception or position sense.

- **Motor nerves** The motor nerves carry impulses away from the brain or spinal cord, to muscles and glands, and produce movement.

The two main parts of the nervous system are the central nervous system and the peripheral nervous system.

11.2 Central Nervous System (CNS)

The central nervous system consists of the brain and spinal cord. The brain contains centers that control involuntary functions such as circulation, temperature regulation, respiration, and impressions from the eyes and ears. It is the processing center of consciousness, emotion, thought, memory, and reasoning.

Major structures of the brain include the following:

- The *cerebrum* is responsible for memory, interpretation of sensations, and voluntary movement.

- The *cerebellum* coordinates voluntary movement, posture, and equilibrium.

- The *medulla* functions as the center for respiration, blood pressure, and cardiac activity. The medulla and its accompanying structures are sometimes called the *brainstem*.

Figure 11.1

The Nervous
System

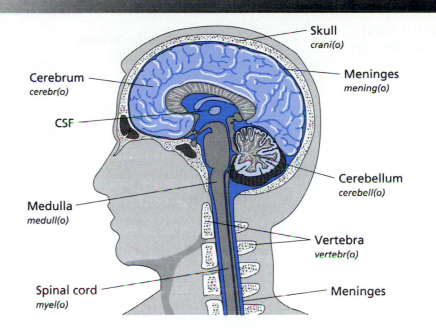

Skull
crani(o)

Cerebrum
cerebr(o)

Meninges
mening(o)

CSF

Cerebellum
cerebell(o)

Medulla
medull(o)

Vertebra
vertebr(o)

Spinal cord
myel(o)

Meninges

Figure 11.1 shows the major structures of the brain and the
protective structures. The spinal cord is found within the spinal
column, surrounded by the vertebrae. It connects to the medulla
and ends about the level of the first lumbar vertebra. The function
of the spinal cord is to relay messages (*impulses*) from the body to
the brain and from the brain to the body.

The brain and spinal cord are surrounded by thin membranes
called the *meninges* (pia mater, arachnoid, and dura mater), which
are protective structures. Within these membranes is the fluid
called *cerebrospinal fluid* (CSF), which serves as a shock absorber. In
Figure 11.2 on page 166, a cross section illustrates the location of the
cord and spinal nerves surrounded by the meninges and vertebra.

Figure 11.2

Spinal Cord
Cross Section

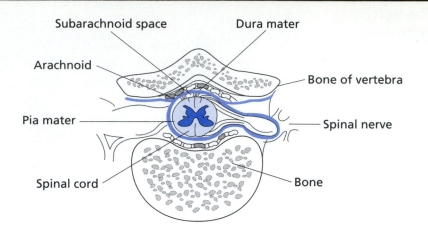

Subarachnoid space   Dura mater

Arachnoid

Bone of vertebra

Pia mater

Spinal nerve

Spinal cord

Bone

11.3   Peripheral Nervous System

The peripheral nervous system involves the cranial nerves (off the brain), spinal nerves (off the spinal cord), and the autonomic (automatic) nerves. It links the CNS and body parts such as the skin, muscles, and internal organs.

- **Cranial nerves** Attached to the undersurface of the brain are the cranial nerves. There are 12 pairs (arranged on the right and left sides of the brain). Each pair has a name and controls impulses mainly in the head and neck region.

- **Spinal nerves** The spinal nerves are attached to the right and the left sides of the spinal cord and exit through openings between the vertebrae. There are 31 pairs, corresponding to their location. (For example, L3-4 means its location is between the third and fourth lumbar vertebrae.) The spinal nerves conduct impulses between parts of the body and the spinal cord.

- **Autonomic nervous system** The autonomic nervous system controls the internal organs and normal functions. It works with adrenaline in times of stress. The functions that are affected are breathing, circulation, digestion, excretion, and hormone secretion.

STYLE TIP

Spinal nerves are labeled using the letter of their location (*C* = cervical, *T* = thoracic, and *L* = lumbar) followed by the appropriate Arabic numeral.

11.4 The Sense Organs

Functions of the sense organs are taste, smell, sight, hearing, and sensation. The eyes and ears are briefly discussed in this unit.

- **The eyes** Each eye is located in the eye socket or *orbit* and is surrounded by bone for protection. Three layers of tissue form the eyeball: the *sclera*, or "white" part of the eye; the *choroid* or middle layer that contains special muscles and blood vessels; and the *retina* or inner layer that contains the cells of vision.

Use Figure 11.3 to locate the following structures within the eye:

- The **conjunctiva**, a thin membrane covering the front of the eyeball and lining the eyelids

- The **cornea**, the transparent covering of the eye overlying the muscular iris, the colored part of the eye

- The **pupil**, a hole in the center of the iris that allows light to enter

- The **lens**, a transparent body that focuses light rays on the retina

- The **cranial nerve** (*optic*), which transmits the impulses to the brain for interpretation (vision)

- The **lacrimal glands** (*tear glands*), placed superiorly and laterally with their ducts and draining into the nose

The extraocular muscles (EOMs) move the eyes in all directions.

Figure 11.3

The Structures of the Eye

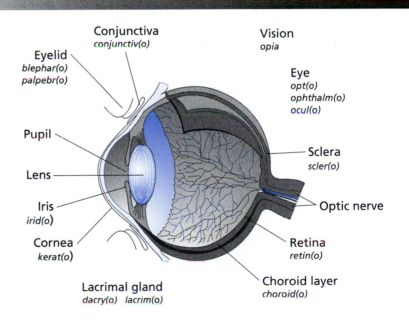

Conjunctiva
conjunctiv(o)

Vision
opia

Eyelid
blephar(o)
palpebr(o)

Eye
opt(o)
ophthalm(o)
ocul(o)

Pupil

Sclera
scler(o)

Lens

Iris
irid(o)

Optic nerve

Cornea
kerat(o)

Retina
retin(o)

Lacrimal gland
dacry(o) lacrim(o)

Choroid layer
choroid(o)

- **The ears** The ears are located in the temporal region of the skull. The external or visible part of the ear is the *pinna*. Extending inward is the *auditory canal*, which is lined with hairs. The lining secretes *cerumen*, which along with the hairs aids in preventing the entrance of foreign substances.

The middle ear is a tiny cavity lined with mucous membrane. The innermost part contains the *ossicles*, which vibrate with sound waves. The *tympanic membrane* (TM), or eardrum, separates the middle ear from the external ear. The *eustachian tube* is a pathway leading from the middle ear to the throat; it functions in equalizing pressure to facilitate vibrations of the tympanic membrane. These vibrations are transmitted to the *labyrinth* (inner ear). The inner ear contains the acoustic nerve for hearing as well as structures that aid in maintaining balance.

Locate the above structures in Figure 11.4.

Figure 11.4

The Structures
of the Ear

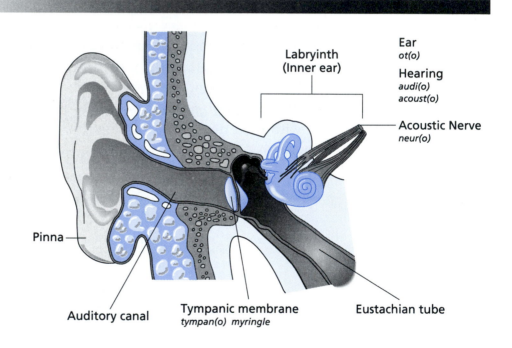

Labryinth
(Inner ear)

Ear
ot(o)

Hearing
audi(o)
acoust(o)

Acoustic Nerve
neur(o)

Pinna

Auditory canal

Tympanic membrane
tympan(o) myringle

Eustachian tube

11.5 Clinical Assessment

The neurologic examination includes questions about headache, syncope, vertigo, pain, paralysis, and the emotional state of the patient.

The eye exam includes the gross general exam, noting that the pupils are equal, round, and reactive to light and accommodation (*PERRLA*). The funduscopic exam checks the retinae and optic disks. The extraocular movements or motions (*EOMs*) check the movement of eye muscles. More definitive tests may include visual fields (central and peripheral vision) and visual acuity.

The examiner tests *tactile* (touch) sensation and two-point discrimination (ability to distinguish two compass points 2 to 3 cm apart), perception of pain (*pinprick*) and temperature, joint position, vibratory sense, coordination (finger-to-nose, heel-to-shin, tandem walk), and gait.

The Romberg test examines coordination. Deep tendon reflexes (DTRs) include the biceps, triceps, brachioradial, knee and ankle jerks, and plantar reflex (Babinski's sign).

The reflexes are graded on a scale of 0 to 4.

Each of the cranial nerves is tested with a specific task the patient is asked to perform (for example, shrugging the shoulders, squinting, or pursing the lips).

11.6 Symptoms and Disease Conditions

KEY *terms* The following symptoms and disease conditions apply to the nervous system. Each term on this list is pronounced at the beginning of the dictation for this chapter. Study the list carefully, practicing pronunciation and building word recognition. Be sure you can spell each term correctly.

TERM	PRONUNCIATION	MEANING
aphasia	(ă-fā′zē-ă)	impaired speech
apraxia	(ă-prak′zē-ă)	inability to perform voluntary movement
astigmatism	(ă-stig′mă-tizm)	warped or distorted image
ataxia	(ă-tak′sē-ă)	inability to coordinate voluntary muscles for movement
blepharitis	(blef′a-rī-tis)	inflammation of eyelid
cataract	(kat′ă-rakt)	loss of transparency of eye lens
cerebrovascular accident (CVA)	(ser′ē-brō-vas′kyū-lăr)	stroke
concussion	(kon-kŭsh′ŭn)	violent jarring of brain
conjunctivitis	(kon-jŭnk-ti-vī′tis)	inflammation of conjunctiva
convulsion	(kon-vŭl′shŭn)	seizure
detached retina		retina pulled away from the choroid
epilepsy	(ep′i-lep′sē)	excessive electrical activity in brain
exophthalmos/exophthalmus	(ek-sof-thal′mos)	bulging eyeballs
focal	(fō′kăl)	located in one area; localized
ganglion	(gang′glē-on)	cystlike swelling
glaucoma	(glaw-kō-mă)	disease characterized by increased intraocular pressure
hematoma	(hē-mă-tō′mă)	localized collection of blood
herpes zoster	(her′pēz zos′ter)	shingles
ischemia	(is-kē′mē-ă)	decreased blood supply
labyrinthitis	(lab′ĭ-rin-thī′tis)	inflammation in inner ear
lightheadedness		dizziness
macular degeneration	(mak′yū-lăr)	deterioration of retina
migraine	(mī′grān)	severe headache
multiple sclerosis	(mŭl′ti-pl sklĕ-rō′sis)	formation of plaque in the brain or spinal cord causing some degree of tremor, paralysis, or speech disturbance
nuchal rigidity	(nū′kăl)	stiff neck
numbness	(nŭm′nes)	absence of feeling
nystagmus	(nis-tag′mŭs)	jerking eye movement
paralysis	(pă-ral′i-sis)	loss of voluntary movement

TERM	PRONUNCIATION	MEANING
paresthesia	(par-es-thē´zē-ă)	abnormal sensation; tingling
Parkinson's disease	(par´kin-son)	shaking or trembling palsy
photophobia	(fō-tō-fō´bē-ă)	sensitivity to light
ptosis	(tō´sis)	downward organ displacement
sciatica	(sī-at´i-kă)	pain in lower back and hip radiating down posterior thigh
sty or stye	(stī)	inflammation of oil gland of eyelid
syncope	(sin´kŏ-pē)	fainting
transient ischemic attack (TIA)	(trans´shĕnt is-kē´mik)	short-term interruption of blood supply to brain; mild stroke
tremor	(trem´er)	involuntary trembling or shaking
vertigo	(ver´ti-go)	feeling as if room is spinning; dizziness
visual acuity	(ă-kyū´i-tē)	sharpness or clearness of sight

11.7 Medical and Surgical Procedures

KEYterms The procedural terms that appear in the dictation for this chapter are described below. Study each term's spelling, pronunciation, and meaning so you are prepared for transcription.

TERM	PRONUNCIATION	MEANING
audiogram	(aw´dē-ō-gram)	hearing test
carotid ultrasound	(ka-rot´id)	image showing blood flow through carotid arteries
cataract extraction	(kat´ă-rakt ek-strak´shŭn)	removal of cataract
CT scan	(C-T-skăn)	imaging to detect abnormalities or mass; use of a dye permits visualization of vessels
electroencephalogram (EEG)	(ēlek´trō-en-sef´ă-lō-gram)	record of brain activity
funduscopy	(fŭn-dŭs´kō-pē)	examine eye interior (eye ground)
intraocular lens implant	(in´tră-ok´yū-lăr)	implanting a new lens
MRI		imaging to detect tissue lesions, particularly in brainstem and spinal cord
tympanogram	(tim´pă-nō-gram)	test the vibrating function of tympanic membranes
visual refraction	(rē-frak´shŭn)	routine eye (acuity) exam

11.8 Medications

The medications that appear in the dictation for this chapter are described below. Study each medication's spelling, pronunciation, and classification.

TERM	PRONUNCIATION	CLASSIFICATION
amitriptyline	(am-i-trip´ti-lēn)	antidepressant
Antivert	(ant´i-vert)	antivertigo
Biaxin	(bī-ak´sin)	antibiotic
Cafergot	(kaf´er-got)	vasoconstrictor
Fluorescein	(flūr-es´ē-in)	dye indicator for corneal trauma
Gantrisin	(gan´tri-sin)	antibiotic
Garamycin	(gar-ă-mī´sin)	antibiotic
Imitrex	(im´i-trex)	antimigraine
Midrin	(mid´ren)	analgesic
phenobarbital	(fē-nō-bar´bi-tahl)	sedative
Pontocaine	(pont´ō-kāin)	anesthetic
Sodium Sulamyd	(sul´ă-mid)	bacteriostatic
sulfacetamide	(sŭl-fă-set´ă-mīd)	bacteriostatic
Valium	(val´ē-ŭm)	antianxiety
Visine	(vī-sēn´)	ocular decongestant

11.9 Related Terms

The following terms appear in the dictation for this chapter. Study the spelling, pronunciation, and meaning of these terms.

TERM	PRONUNCIATION	MEANING
basilar	(bas´i-lăr)	base of a structure, such as the brain
embedded or imbedded	(em-bed´ed)	fixed in surrounding tissue
gaze	(gāz)	look steadily
hertz (Hz)	(herts´)	unit of frequency
ophthalmology	(of-thal-mol´ō-jē)	branch of medicine concerned with diagnosis and treatment of eye diseases
otolarnygology	(o´to-lar-ing-gol´ŏ-jē)	branch of medicine concerned with diagnosis and treatment of ears, nose, and throat

TERM	PRONUNCIATION	MEANING
punctate	(pŭngk´tāt)	tiny specks
sensorium	(sen-sō´rē-ŭm)	intellectual functions
sphincter	(sfingk´ter)	muscle that controls size of an opening
variant	(vār´ē-ant)	different from standard
vascular	(vas´kyū-lăr)	pertaining to a vessel

11.10 Build Your Editing Skills

In this section, you will gain the skills you need to correctly transcribe medical documents.

Selecting the Right Word

The words listed here are often confused in transcription because they sound alike when dictated but have different meanings. Study the words carefully so that you will be able to select the correct term according to the context of the dictation.

TERM/PRONUNCIATION	MEANING	EXAMPLE
antepyretic (an´te-pī-ret´ik)	before fever; before the reaction to shock	An antepyretic condition for this disease is the sweats.
antipyretic (an´tē-pī-ret´ik)	reducing fever; agent to reduce fever	Children's Tylenol is an effective OTC antipyretic.
chord	combination of musical notes	The student played a chord on the piano.
cord	long ropelike structure; to become stringlike	The spinal cord was damaged from the injury.
regimen (rej´i-men)	program outlining therapeutic course such as diet, exercise, and so forth for restoring or maintaining health	The patient's regimen for diabetes included wearing a medical ID bracelet.
regiment (red´ja-ment)	a military unit; to render useless or to use overt control	The school was too regimented for the doctor's family.

Using the Correct Punctuation

Medical transcriptionists use correct punctuation when preparing medical documents. Review the following punctuation guidelines. (The basic medical transcription guidelines are in Appendix A.)

GUIDELINE

Roman numerals are preferred for cranial nerves, but Arabic numerals are also acceptable. Ordinals for cranial nerves are preferred to be written out, but also are acceptable in numeric form. Be consistent and follow the physician's preference.

Enumerate listings as much as possible. In sentence format, enclose numbers in parentheses.

For lists, the block style is preferred with entries aligning at the left margin. Do not place numbers in parentheses. Capitalize the first letter of each entry, and end each entry with a period.

EXAMPLE

Cranial nerves II-XII were consistent with the results from 3 years ago. *or* Cranial nerves 2-12 were consistent with the results from 3 years ago.

The fifth cranial nerve was not tested. *or* The 5th cranial nerve was not tested.

Do not forget to include the following items with your research paper: (1) bibliography, (2) cover sheet, and (3) one extra copy that will not be returned to you.

FINAL DIAGNOSES
1. Diabetes mellitus.
2. Arteriosclerotic heart disease.
3. Senile dementia.

Name _____ Date _____

Exercise 11.1 Building Your Medical Vocabulary

Directions Define the following word forms.

Term	**Definition**
1. adeno	_____
2. audio	_____
3. blepharo	_____
4. cephalo	_____
5. cerebro	_____
6. conjunctivo	_____
7. cranio	_____
8. encephalo	_____
9. kerato	_____
10. dacryo	_____
11. lacrimo	_____
12. meningo	_____
13. myringo or tympano	_____
14. neuro	_____
15. oculo or ophthalmo	_____
16. oto	_____
17. peri	_____
18. retino	_____
19. -phasia	_____
20. photo	_____
21. -algia	_____
22. -esthesia	_____
23. -itis	_____
24. -metry	_____
25. -opia	_____
26. -pathy	_____
27. -osis	_____
28. -scopy	_____

Exercise 11.2 Matching Symptoms and Disease Descriptions

Directions Match the symptom or disease in Column 2 with the definition in Column 1.

Column 1	Column 2
____ 1. tingling sensation	**a.** analgesia
____ 2. involuntary eye movement	**b.** anesthesia
____ 3. spinning sensation	**c.** aphasia
____ 4. cloudy lens	**d.** ataxia
____ 5. sensitivity to light	**e.** cataract
____ 6. infected oil gland of eyelid	**f.** convulsion
____ 7. drooping of eyelid	**g.** focal
____ 8. poor ability to talk	**h.** glaucoma
____ 9. loss of sensation	**i.** ischemia
____ 10. poor coordination when walking	**j.** nystagmus
____ 11. fainting	**k.** paresthesia
____ 12. located in one area	**l.** photophobia
____ 13. poor blood supply	**m.** ptosis
____ 14. seizure	**n.** syncope
____ 15. insensitivity to pain	**o.** stye
____ 16. increased intraocular pressure	**p.** vertigo

Exercise 11.3 Working with Abbreviations

Directions Provide the meanings of the following abbreviations.

1. EEG _____

2. TM _____

3. CSF _____

4. PERRLA _____

5. DTR _____

6. EOM _____

Exercise 11.4 Applying Your Editing Skills

Directions Circle the correct term in the following statements.

1. The spermatic *chord / cord* was intact.

2. The patient was given an *antepyretic / antipyretic* for the fever.

3. The *regimen / regiment* included medication, stress management, and attendance at support group meetings.

4. Diagnoses are *1) tonsillitis, 2) sinusitis, and 3) bronchitis. / (1) tonsillitis, (2) sinusitis, and (3) bronchitis.*

5. Cranial nerves *2-XII / 2-12 / II-12* are intact.

6. ASSESSMENT   ASSESSMENT

   1. Anxiety.   or   *(1) Anxiety.*

   2. Hematochezia.   *(2) Hematochezia.*

7. The physician prescribed the *antepyretic / antipyretic*, naproxen, for the elderly patient with fever, chills, and nausea.

8. The physician prescribed a *regimen / regiment* for the patient's panic disorder including behavior therapy and supportive psychotherapy.

9. After delivery of the infant, *chord / cord* blood was obtained.

10. The *sixth / 6* cranial nerve needs to be retested.

HINTS FOR TRANSCRIPTION

Before you begin the transcription for this chapter, be sure you know the following items.

Cranial Nerves

Roman numberals are generally used to describe the twelve cranial nerves.

> Cranial nerves II-XII are grossly intact.

> *Note:* Cranial nerve I is the olfactory for smell and is generally not tested, except in an extensive exam of all the cranial nerves.

Reflex Grades

A reflex of 0 would indicate no response; 1+ is low normal; 2+ is average or normal; 3+ is brisker than normal; and 4+ is indicative of a disease process.

Visual Acuity Measurement

Visual acuity is measured at 20 feet. Thus the first number is always 20; the second number will vary according to the vision as measured on a standard scale. Therefore, 20/20 is considered normal; 20/200 is ability to see only the largest letter on the vision chart.

Hearing Measurement

Hearing is measured from 125 or 250 to 8000 Hz. Hearing loss is measured in decibels (dB).

MEDICAL DOCUMENT TRANSCRIPTION

You are now ready to transcribe the dictation for Chapter 11.

The dictation for this chapter is by Lynn Solinski, MD. Remember to properly identify each report in the upper right corner.

> Chapter 11, Item 1
> Your Name
> Current Date

---

11 TRANSCRIPTION CHECKOFF SHEET

Use the transcription checkoff sheet to record your work and track your progress as a medical transcriptionist.

DOCTOR DICTATING Lynn Solinski, MD
TYPE OF DICTATION Chart notes, history and physical, and letters
DATE OF TRANSCRIPTION April 24, 20—

Item Number	Patient	Date Started	Date Completed	Grade/ Number of Errors
11.1	Julia Liberstrom			
11.2	Andrew Brewster			
11.3	Letter to Peter Saakara, MD RE: Marsha Dahlheimer			
11.4	Jared Carlos			
11.5	Peter Colburn, MD RE: Donovan Westrum			
11.6	Arnold Stronovich			
11.7	Lia Jen Chambers			
11.8	Richard Lighttree			
11.9	Heather Sherman			
11.10	Tamara Neubauer			
11.11	Timothy Blesi			

TRANSCRIPTION TEST 4

After the Chapter 11 transcription has been corrected and returned to you for review, you are ready to take the fourth transcription test. Obtain the testing information from your instructor.

Case Studies

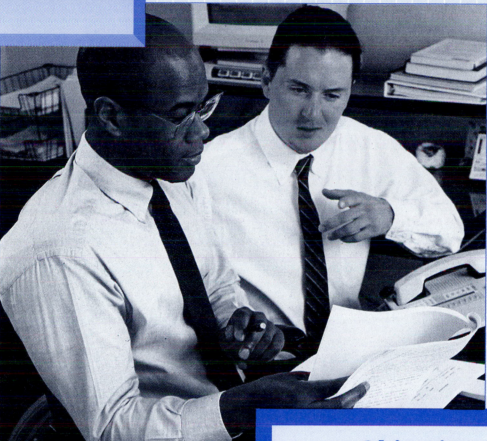

Documents concerning a patient's health care must be transcribed in a timely fashion by skilled medical transcriptionists. *In what order should documents be placed in the patient's medical record?*

Objectives

After completing this chapter, you will be able to

1. Review the medical record.
2. Describe the sequence of the documents in a patient's medical record.
3. Review the procedure for correcting an error in transcription.

In this final chapter of the text-workbook, two case studies are followed as transcription is performed. To successfully complete this chapter, you must apply the knowledge and skill you have gained in studying the previous chapters. You should also observe the types of documents and the reasons they are included in the patients' records in the case studies.

Case Study 1: Dictation on patient Rolland Severson

Type of Report	Dictating physician	Transcription date
Chart note	John Blackburn, MD	April 27, 20—
History and physical examination	Lee Kim, MD	April 28, 20—
Letter	Lee Kim, MD	May 5, 20—

Case Study 2: Dictation on patient Naomi Geiger

Type of Report	Dictating physician	Transcription date
Chart note	Debra Litman, MD	April 29, 20—
History and physical examination	Lynn Solinski, MD	April 30, 20—
Chart note	Debra Litman, MD	May 13, 20—

As soon as you are ready, begin the transcription for Chapter 12.

Appendix A: Basic Medical Transcription Guidelines

Review the following guidelines and apply them to your transcription.

1. Use commas to
   a. Set off nonessential words and phrases.
      Dr. Jones, a first-year resident, is on call.
      Janice, who was hired last month, will attend next week's conference.
   b. Set off introductory clauses or phrases.
      After the cast was applied, the x-ray showed the fracture to be in good alignment.
      If so, the physician will have to leave an hour before closing.
   c. Separate the year in a complete date. Do **not** use commas when only the month and year are presented. (*Note:* Do **not** use numerals for dates in text material; e.g., The surgery is scheduled for 11/01/03.)
      The surgery is scheduled for Tuesday, May 1, 20—.
      The patient was last seen in May 2000 for an ultrasound.
   d. Separate degrees, titles, etc., following names.
      The patient was referred to Phil Stevens, PhD, for psychological testing.
   e. Separate items in a series.
      The sponge, needle, and instrument counts were correct.
   f. Separate independent sentences connected with a conjunction.
      Mrs. Tina Roe called last hour, and she still insists on seeing the physician today.
   g. Set off direct address in a sentence.
      Set the chart on the desk, Janis, and take the new dictation tape with you.
   h. Separate equal adjectives (modifiers).
      The patient is a well-nourished, well-developed female.
      The 15-year-old Caucasian male has brain cancer.
      (The adjective "15-year-old" modifies both Caucasian and male; therefore, no comma is used.)
   i. Place commas and periods inside quotation marks.
      The patient states that he feels "fuzzy in the head," and he needs medication for this symptom.
   j. Use a comma to indicate missing words.
      Chest x-ray, normal. (Chest x-ray was normal.)
   k. Use a comma to separate parts of an inverted diagnosis.
      Ankle sprain, left.
2. Use semicolons to
   a. Separate related independent clauses (sentences) without a conjunction.
      The surgery was scheduled for 4 p.m.; it lasted 4 hours.

    b. Set off independent clauses that already contain one or more commas and have a conjunction, if a misreading might result.

> *If, following the call, the appointment has been made, Janet can leave at 9:30 p.m.; but if the appointment has not been made, she needs to leave right away.*

    c. Separate a transitional word or phrase that begins an independent sentence, such as *therefore, however, in fact, namely, thus*, etc., from another independent sentence.

> *The physician will be 2 hours late; however, there are no patients scheduled until this afternoon.*

    d. Separate items in a series when the items have commas.

> *The physician has lectures scheduled in St. Paul, Minnesota; Fargo, North Dakota; and Des Moines, Iowa.*

    e. Place semicolons outside of quotation marks.

> *The patient said, "I will obtain my medical records"; she did not bring them to the office.*

3. Use a colon to

    a. Introduce a list, series, or enumeration.

> *The patient complains of the following symptoms: dizziness, lightheadedness, and palpitations.*
> *The patient was instructed to do the following:*
> > *1. Follow a low-fat, low cholesterol diet.*
> > *2. Exercise 3 times a week.*
> > *3. Retest cholesterol in 3 months.*

    b. Separate hours and minutes.

> *The surgery is scheduled to begin at 12:30 p.m.*

    c. Introduce an example, a rule, or a principle.

> *We have only one choice: immediate surgery.*

4. Use capital letters in the following situations:

    a. Emphasize allergies in full capital letters. (*Note:* An alternative method is to use boldface.)

> *The patient was ALLERGIC TO PENICILLIN.*
> *ALLERGIES: Penicillin.*

    b. Do **not** capitalize common nouns designating rooms, such as operating room or emergency room.
Capitalize the official names of designated rooms.

> *The patient was seen in the intensive care unit.*
> *(Note: The patient was seen in the ICU.)*
> *The patient is scheduled for the operating room in an hour.*
> *The patient was sent to Recovery Room C at 9 a.m.*
> *The meeting will take place in the Viking Room.*

    c. Do **not** capitalize medical specialties or variations of specialties.

> *The patient was referred to cardiology.*
> *The cardiologist sent the patient back to the family practice physician.*

d. Capitalize trade and brand names but do not capitalize generic names; for example, Tylenol #3, pHisoHex, and Cardizem, but alcohol, catgut, and aspirin.

e. Capitalize races, peoples, religions, and languages but generally not color designations such as *black* or *white* when they refer to race (Caucasian, African American, Jewish, Hispanic, Mexican American, English, etc.).

> *The patient is a well-developed, well-nourished Caucasian male.*
> *The patient is a well-developed, well-nourished white female.*
> *The 31-year-old black patient was discharged yesterday.*

f. Use full capitalization for headings and subheadings in the medical document.

> *GENITOURINARY*
> *Exam will be completed next month.*

5. Use a hyphen to
   a. Connect the elements of compound adjectives that appear before nouns.

   > *She had a low-grade temperature. (Note: Her temperature was low grade.)*
   > *This was a well-developed Asian male.*
   > *There was a 5-cm lesion on the left side.*

   b. Form **self** compounds.

   > *The patient was self-employed.*

   c. Look up compound nouns in a current dictionary to determine whether they are hyphenated or closed up. Use two separate nonhyphenated words for two-word verbs.

   > *The patient is scheduled for a follow-up visit.*
   > *The patient's checkup was delayed.*
   > *The patient will follow up with hematology.*

   d. Join a single letter to a word to form a coined compound word.

   > *The patient had a T-cell abnormality. (Note: We will measure the patient's T cells.)*
   > *The x-ray results will be sent to the office.*

   e. Insert a hyphen between a prefix and a capitalized word such as non-Hodgkin or mid-March.

6. Use abbreviations as follows:
   a. Use published/medical abbreviations.

   > *The mole is 1.25 cm in circumference with irregular borders.*

   b. Use proper abbreviations for transcribing medication administration times.

   > *The patient was placed on Augmentin 125 mg t.i.d. x 5 days.*
   > *A prescription for tetracycline 500 mg q.i.d. was given to the patient.*

(*Note:* Always keep units of measurement on same line.)

  c. Do not abbreviate the diagnosis, conclusion, or procedural/operative title in medical documents. Nondisease-related words in the diagnostic or procedural titles may be abbreviated.

  > *DIAGNOSIS*
  > *End stage renal disease.* (**not** ESRD)
  > *OPERATION*
  > *Excise 0.5-cm polyp from right naris.*

  d. Spell out a word if the abbreviation could be misunderstood.

  > *The patient has no history of a cancer problem.* (CA could mean calcium, cancer, coronary artery, etc.)

  e. Do **not** abbreviate beats per minute.

  > *Pulse was 72 beats per minute.*

  f. Use lowercase letters with periods for a.m. and p.m. (preferred style). Spell out even times when a.m., p.m., or o'clock is not used.

  > *The next available appointment is for 10 a.m.*
  > *The patient will be seen at three.*

7. Use numbers as follows:
  a. Spell out numbers at the beginning of a sentence, or recast the sentence.

  > *Ten milligrams was given to the patient.*
  > *The nurse gave 10 mg to the patient.*

  b. Use Arabic numbers with technical measurements.

  > *A #14 Foley catheter was inserted.*
  > *A No. 4 Foley catheter was inserted.*
  > *The surgeon suggested 5- to 6-inch elastic stays.*

  c. Express ages and other numbers in figures when used as significant statistics or as technical measurements.

  > *This 5-year-old boy has had cold symptoms for the past 2 weeks.*
  > *The 5 1/2-month-old child was not left unattended.*
  > *The patient was given 10 tablets.*
  > *The patient was prescribed Paxil 20 mg q.d., #60.*

  d. Spell out ordinal numbers and single fractions (preferred style).

  > *The patient was discharged on the fifth postoperative day.*
  > *Next, one-third of the abdomen was prepped.*

  e. Use roman numerals for cranial nerves, ECG leads, EEG leads, clotting factors, and noncounting listings (preferred style).

  > *The exam found that the cranial nerves II-XII were intact.*
  > *The patient had stage II carcinoma.*
  > *The patient had type II diabetes mellitus.*

  f. Use Arabic numbers with grades.

  > *The patient had a grade 2 systolic ejection murmur.*

g. Insert a zero in front of the decimal point when a decimal is less than a whole number.

> *The patient's prescription was changed to 0.125 mg.*

h. Enumerate listings as much as possible.

> *DIAGNOSES*
> 1. *Right otitis media.*
> 2. *Laryngitis.*
> 3. *Pharyngitis.*
>
> *The diagnoses were (1) right otitis media, (2) laryngitis, and (3) pharyngitis.*

i. Do **not** repeat units of measure in a series.

> *The patient was given 5, 10, and 20 cc.*

8. Use symbols when transcribing numbers or abbreviations. Some common examples are shown below.

Heard	*Keyboarded*
used two oh chromic catgut	*used 2-0 chromic catgut*
two by point five millimeter	*2.0 x 0.5 mm*
number two oh silk	*#2-0 silk or 2-0 silk*
one point two percent	*1.2%*
pulses are two plus	*pulses are 2+*
blood pressure one hundred twenty over eighty	*Blood pressure: 120/80*
fifty-five milligrams percent	*55 mg%*
diluted one to one hundred	*diluted 1:100*
ninety-nine degrees Fahrenheit	*99°F*
the plane was raised ten degrees	*The plane was raised 10 degrees.* (Note: Spell out degrees in expressing angles.)
at a minus two station	*at a –2 station*
medication times three days	*medication x 3 days*
one hundred milligrams per hour	*100 mg/h*
normal "es" one and "es" two	*normal S_1 and S_2* *normal S1 and S2* *normal S-1 and S-2*
one hundred milligrams per teaspoon	*100 mg/teaspoon*
ten to fifteen wbcs	*10-15 wbc's* *10-15 WBCs*
two to four plus	*2 to 4+*

9. Follow proper guidelines for letters and memorandums. Use a reference manual.

10. Consult a reference manual about questionable punctuation, capitalization, and grammar.

11. Use an acceptable and approved format for each medical document.

Abbreviations for Weights and Measures (medication dosages and lab values)

length or thickness

centimeter	cm
meter	m
millimeter	mm

weight

grain	gr
gram	g (preferred) or gm
kilogram	kg
milligram	mg
microgram	mcg

volume

cubic centimeter	cc
liter	L
milliliter	mL (liquid volume)
unit	U

Abbreviations Designating Times and Methods

a.c.	before a meal
b.i.d.	twice a day
h	hour
IM	intramuscular
IV	intravenous
n.p.o.	nothing by mouth
p.c.	after meals
p.o.	per os (by mouth)
p.r.n.	as desired or as needed
q.	every
q.i.d.	four times a day
q.2h.	every two hours
q.d.	every day
q.h.	every hour
q.o.d.	every other day
stat or STAT	immediately
subq/subcu	subcutaneous
t.i.d.	three times a day

Abbreviations Related to Chart Notes

BP	blood pressure
CC	chief complaint
ER	emergency room
FH	family history
F/U	follow-up
GI	gastrointestinal
GU	genitourinary
GYN	gynecology
H&P	history and physical
HPI	history of present illness
HS	hour of sleep
ICU	intensive care unit
n.p.o	nothing per os (by mouth)
OB	obstetrics
PE	physical exam
PERRLA	pupils equal, round, reactive to light and accommodation
PMH	past medical history
p.r.n.	as necessary or as desired
R/O	rule out
ROS	review of systems
SH	social history
S/P	status post
STAT	right now
TPR	temperature, pulse, respirations
UA	urinalysis
VS	vital signs
WBC	white blood count
wbc	white blood cells

Brief Forms

Brief forms (short forms) are accepted forms of full words that are not abbreviated. Generally, they are derived from common usage. Some examples are listed below.

chem profile	chemistry profile
cysto	cystoscopy
echo	echocardiogram
exam	examination
flex sig	flexible sigmoidoscopy
flu	influenza
Pap smear	Papanicolaou smear
pro-time	prothrombin time
rehab	rehabilitation
sed rate	sedimentation rate
temp	temperature

Appendix C: Drug Classifications

Drugs and medicines are classified according to their use in the body. Some common classifications are shown in the following list:

analgesic	gives pain relief	**cardiotonics**	affects heart action
anesthetic	causes loss of sensation	**contraceptive**	prevents conception or pregnancy
antacid	neutralizes acidity, especially in the GI tract	**cortisone and steroids**	influence metabolism, inflammation, and physiologic stress
antianxiety	relieves emotional tension	**decongestant**	decreases congestion or swelling in respiratory tract
antiarrhythmic	regulates irregular heart rhythm	**disinfectant**	destroys bacteria on objects; not used on living tissue
antibiotic	kills living microorganisms that cause infection		
anticoagulant	prevents blood clotting	**diuretic**	increases urine output
anticonvulsant	prevents convulsions and seizures	**emetic**	causes vomiting
		expectorant	aids in expelling mucus from respiratory tract
antidepressant	relieves depression		
antidiabetic	treats diabetes	**glucocorticoid and cortico-steroids**	influence metabolism and reduce inflammation
antidiarrheal	relieves or corrects diarrhea		
antidote	counteracts or neutralizes a poison	**hypolipidemic**	lowers blood cholesterol
		keratolytic	assists in loosening horny layer of skin
antiemetic	reduces vomiting		
antihistamine	treats allergy symptoms	**laxative**	aids in having a bowel movement
antihypertensive	lowers blood pressure		
anti-inflammatory	reduces inflammation	**miotic**	causes pupil of eye to contract
antimicrobial	destroys microorganisms		
antineoplastic	treats cancers	**mydriatic**	causes pupil of eye to dilate
antipruritic	relieves itching		
antipsychotic	treats psychotic (out-of-touch-with-reality) disorders	**narcotic**	relieves pain or causes sleep; addictive
		NSAID	nonsteroidal anti-inflammatory drug
antipyretic	reduces fever		
antiseptic	stops growth of microorganisms	**scabicide**	destroys scabies
		sedative	exerts tranquilizing, soothing effect
antitussive	relieves cough		
antivertigo	relieves dizziness	**stimulant**	increases activity
antiviral	weakens a virus	**vaccine**	causes resistance to specific disease
anxiolytic	relieves anxiety		
bacteriostatic	inhibits growth of bacteria	**vasoconstrictor**	causes blood vessels to constrict
		vasodilator	causes vessels to dilate
bronchodilator	dilates bronchial tubes		

Alkaline Phosphatase   (al´kă-lĭn fos´fă-tās)

Alkaline phosphatase (alk phos) is an enzyme found primarily in the liver and in bone. The test is useful in diagnosing or monitoring the progress of liver disease, medications that are toxic to the liver, and bone diseases.

Normal range: 20 to 90 IU/L

Amylase   (am´il-ăs)

Amylase is a digestive enzyme produced in the pancreas, salivary glands, and liver. Normally, very little amylase is found in the blood or urine. Serum levels are used to evaluate pancreatitis; urine amylase is performed on a 2-hour or 24-hour specimen.

Normal serum level: 60 to 160 Somogyl U/L

Bilirubin   (bil-i-rū´bin)

Bilirubin is a pigmented by-product of hemoglobin breakdown that is carried to the liver for further metabolism and then excreted through the bile ducts into the intestine, giving the stool its normal brown color. It is called *indirect* before being acted on by the liver, and it is called *direct* after being metabolized by the liver. The *total bilirubin* combines both of these measurements; if this is ab-normally high, the individual determinations are made. Abnormalities in bilirubin may be due to liver disease, infectious mononucleosis, gallbladder disease, or blood disease. It may be measured in serum or urine.

Normal serum level: direct, less than 0.3 mg/dl;
indirect, 0.1 to 1.0 mg/dl;
total bilirubin, 0.1 to 1.2 mg/dl (1 to 12 in newborns)

BUN (blood urea nitrogen)

Urea is an end product of protein breakdown. It is formed in the liver, found in the blood in the form of urea nitrogen, and excreted in the urine by the kidneys. BUN is a test for kidney function.

Normal value: 8 to 23 mg/dl

Cholesterol   *(kō-les´ter-ol)*

Cholesterol is a fatty substance (lipid) found in body tissue. It is an essential building block of cell membranes, bile acids, and sex hormones. High levels are associated with the development of coronary artery disease. Cholesterol attaches to proteins in complexes called *lipoproteins* and travels through the bloodstream. The LDL (low-density lipoprotein), or *bad cholesterol*, forms deposits in arterial walls. The HDL (high-density lipoprotein),or *good cholesterol*, may help protect people from coronary artery disease.

Average value is 150 to 200 mg% with the following:
HDL normal, less than 130;
LDL normal, greater than 60; and
total cholesterol to HDL ratio of 3.4

Complete Blood Count (CBC)

This may include 7 or 8 different tests, including the following:

Hematocrit measures the portion of blood volume that is made up of red cells. It is commonly used to test for anemia.

Normal values: women, 37% to 47%; men, 40% to 54%

Hemoglobin is the iron-containing protein found in the red blood cells that carries oxygen to the body tissues. It is a test for anemia.

Normal values: women, 12 to 16 gm/dl; men, 14 to 18 gm/dl

Red blood cell count (RBC) These cells carry oxygen to body tissues and return waste products to the lungs. This is also a test for anemia.

Normal values: women, 4.2 to 5.4 million/cu mm;
men, 4.6 to 6.2 million/cu mm

White blood cell count (WBC) and **differential** The white cells fight infection. Increases in WBCs indicate infection; decreases indicate loss of ability to fight infection. There are several types of white cells, each with a specific function. They include *neutrophils* (PMNs or polys), *bands* (stabs), *lymphocytes* (lymphs), *monocytes* (monos), *eosinophils* (eos), and *basophils*.

Normal values: WBC, 5000 to 10,000; PMNs, 47% to 77%;
bands, 0% to 3%; lymphs, 16% to 43%; monos, 0.5% to 10%;
eos, 0.3% to 7%; basophils, 0.3% to 2%

Platelets These thrombocytes are important in blood clotting and may be evaluated before surgery to diagnose blood diseases, to assess chemotherapy, and to monitor some forms of drug therapy.

Normal values: 150,000 to 400,000

Creatinine (krē-at´i-nēn)

Creatinine is a waste substance from the blood filtered by the kidneys and excreted in the urine. It can be measured in the blood or urine. It is a measurement of kidney function.

Normal serum creatinine: 0.6 to 1.2 mg/dl
Creatinine clearance (urine): women, 87 to 107;
men, 107 to 139 ml/minute

Electrolytes (serum) (ē-lek´trō-līts)

Chloride is a mineral involved in water balance and acid-base balance of body fluids. Abnormalities may cause muscle spasms, breathing abnormalities, weakness, and even coma.

Normal value: 95 to 103 mEq/L

Potassium is a mineral that helps maintain water balance in the cells and is necessary for electrical conduction in nerves and muscles, including the heart. Deficiencies may occur in diabetic acidosis, liver disease, severe burns, excessive use of diuretics, prolonged vomiting, and inadequate potassium intake.

Normal value: 3.8 to 5.0 mEq/L

Sodium is involved in water balance, acid-base balance, and transmission of nerve impulses. Levels depend on the amount of salt and fluid in the diet, fluid losses, and various hormones. The kidneys play a role in excretion and maintenance of salt balance. Abnormalities occur as a result of dehydration, edema, and kidney disorders and may result in agitation, weakness, and confusion.

Normal value: 136 to 142 mEq/L

Bicarbonate (HCO_3) is a buffer that keeps blood from becoming too acid. Much of the bicarbonate is formed through respiration, and the level is regulated by the kidneys. The levels are affected by severe vomiting or diarrhea, excessive intake of antacids, poisoning or other overdoses, diuretics, or difficulty in breathing. Bicarbonate levels are watched closely in disorders of the kidneys or the lungs.

Normal value: vary from 21 to 28 mEq/L

Glucose (glu´kōs)

Glucose is the primary energy source for body tissues. It can be measured in serum or urine. The test may be used to diagnose hypoglycemia or hyperglycemia. (However, many factors interfere with the test.) This test measures the glucose at one particular moment.

Fasting blood sugar: 70 to 110 mg/dl
Two-hour postprandial blood sugar: 120 to 150 mg/dl

Glucose tolerance test (GTT) measures the body's response to a large dose of concentrated sugar over a period of several hours.

Glycohemoglobin (glycosylated hemoglobin or Alc) measures the percentage of hemoglobin molecules that have sugar molecules attached to them. This reflects the blood sugar levels over the preceding 3 to 4 months and is useful in indicating diabetic control.

Normal value: 3 to 6%

Accu-Chek™ is one method of checking the blood glucose level at home.

Clinistix is a test for excretion of sugar in the urine. The test paper should register negative; 1+ to 4+ indicates that glucose is spilling into the urine and is frequently a finding in uncontrolled diabetes.

Mono Test
(heterophil test, mono spot test) (mon´ō)

Mononucleosis is a disease caused by the Epstein-Barr virus. There are two tests: The spot test is a screening test and is read as negative or positive. If positive, the heterophil test can be performed. A positive heterophil or one reported as a ratio greater than 1:224 suggests mononucleosis.

Prothrombin Time (Pro-time) (prō-throm´bin)

Prothrombin is one of a dozen factors necessary for blood clotting. This test measures the blood's ability to clot. An insufficient amount of prothrombin means that it takes longer than normal time for the blood to clot. This may be caused by liver disease, bile duct problem, or medication. The test is performed to monitor oral anticoagulant therapy.

Values are given in seconds, normal (the control) being 11.0 to 12.5 seconds; when a person is on anticoagulant therapy, the value should be about 1.5 to 2 times greater than the control time. The INR (international normalized ratio) is usually maintained around 2. The INR has been introduced to standardize anticoagulant therapy. It is a ratio equation utilizing patient and control pro-times and will replace the more variable pro-time.

Thyroid Function Tests (thī´royd)

TSH is the thyroid-stimulating hormone. T3 and T4 are iodine-containing hormones. These tests are performed to evaluate thyroid function.

Normal value: T3, uptake 25% to 38%; T4, 5 to 11 mcg/dl;

TSH, 0.35 to 7 mU/L

Transaminase
(trans-am´i-nās)

SGOT/AST (aspartate aminotransferase) is an enzyme found mainly in the liver and heart muscle and released into the bloodstream when either of these organs is damaged. The test may be useful in diagnosing and monitoring the progress of disease in either of these organs. Many drugs can cause liver injury, which results in an elevation of this enzyme.

Normal value: 10 to 40 IU/L

SGPT/ALT (alanine aminotransferase) is an enzyme found primarily in the liver and released into the bloodstream as a result of liver damage.

Normal value: 10 to 30 U/ml

Uric Acid
(yūr´ik)

Uric acid is a by-product of body cell function as well as metabolism of certain foods. Uric acid may build up in the body in certain diseases such as gout or kidney disease. It may be measured in the blood or the urine.

Normal serum value: women, 2.7 to 7.3; men, 4 to 8.5 mg/dl

Urinalysis (UA)
(yū-ri-nal´i-sis)

The routine urinalysis (dipstick) gives information about nearly every organ in the body. It consists of visual examination (color and clarity)—urine should be pale or straw yellow and clear; specific gravity (concentration) 1.006 to 1.030; acidity (pH 4.6 to 8.0); chemical tests (glucose, ketones, protein, hemoglobin, bilirubin, and urobilinogen). Examination under the microscope indicates red cells, white cells, bacteria, casts, crystals, and miscellaneous substances if they are present.

Throat Culture

Many organisms produce sore throats. The organism of most concern is the Group A Beta-hemolytic Streptococci (Group A strep) because they can spread to the kidneys or to the heart valves. Cultures are "set up" for 24 hours and then read.

Rapid Strep test gives an immediate response as negative or positive, but if negative and clinical signs indicate a more severe infection, probably a culture will be done for definitive diagnosis.

Heart Attack Enzymes

Testing of three enzymes (CPK, AST, LDH) may be useful in confirming a heart attack. These enzymes leak out of damaged muscle, and there is an elevation in their amounts in the blood. They are frequently drawn on consecutive days (serially). These studies are performed when a heart attack is suspected and aid in that diagnosis.

Cardiac Studies

Electrocardiogram is a graphic recording of electrical activity generated by the heart. It is useful in detecting rhythm, size, and position of heart chambers; muscle inflammation; and abnormalities in minerals that control the electrical activity. It is also used to monitor drugs that affect the heart and to check the function of artificial pacemakers. ECGs are taken at rest.

Cardiac catheterization and **Coronary angiogram** is a procedure in which a catheter is introduced into the heart to determine the severity and location of blocked arteries of the heart, impairment of the valves, and ability of the heart to effectively pump blood. Angiography may be done on other vessels throughout the body.

Ambulatory (Holter) monitoring records heart activity over a 24-hour period.

Exercise ECG (stress test, treadmill test, and exercise tolerance test). This ECG is taken while the patient walks on a treadmill.

Echocardiogram (cardiac echo) shows sound waves (echoes) that are used to evaluate the size, shape, and motion of the heart. It may be used to evaluate abnormal heart sounds, an enlarged heart, palpitations, or blood clots thought to be from the heart.

Computerized Imaging Studies

Magnetic resonance imaging (MRI) uses radio waves to create a magnetic field. Computers process the signals to produce an image. The MRI is used to pinpoint size and location of tumors and diagnose neck and back pain as well as liver and abdominal disease, blood flow in vessels, infections, and eye abnormalities.

Computerized tomography (CT scan) is a study accomplished with a rotating scanner that sends beams of radiation through a specific body area. A computer assembles the beams (image slices) to reveal a detailed image. The scan is used to detect cancer, spinal cord injury, pediatric conditions, and trauma.

Ultrasound sends high-frequency sound waves into the body from a hand-held transducer pressed against the skin. The sound waves echo back from fluid and tissue into a computer that measures them and displays a picture. This test is primarily used to evaluate abdominal and pelvic conditions (gallbladder and pancreas, ovaries, uterus, cysts, tumors, and fetus).

Medical Word Books

Sloane, Sheila B. and Margaret Biblis. *Medical Abbreviations & Eponyms*, 2nd ed. W. B. Saunders Company, 1997.

Drake, Ellen and Sloane, Sheila B. *Sloane's Medical Word Book*, 4th ed. W. B. Saunders Company, 2001.

Stedman's Abbreviations, Acronyms, and Symbols, 2nd ed. Williams & Wilkins, 1999.

Stedman's Alternative Medicine Words. Williams & Wilkins, 2000.

Stedman's Equipment Words, 3rd ed. Williams & Wilkins, 2001.

Stedman's Plus Spellchecker 2001 (CD-ROM). Williams & Wilkins, 2001.

Dictionaries

English dictionaries:

Webster's Third New International Dictionary, Unabridged. Merriam-Webster, Inc., 1993. CD-ROM, 2000.

Medical dictionaries:

Dorland's Illustrated Medical Dictionary, 29th ed. W. B. Saunders Company, 2000.

Miller-Keane Encyclopedia & Dictionary of Medicine, Nursing & Allied Health, 6th ed. W. B. Saunders Company, 1997.

Stedman's Medical Dictionary, Illustrated, 27th ed. Williams & Wilkins, 2000.

Drug Books

Drake, Ellen, and Randy Drake. *Saunders Pharmaceutical Word Book, 2001.* W. B. Saunders Company, 2000.

Physicians' Desk Reference, 2001, 55th ed. Medical Economics, 2001.

Physicians' Desk Reference for Nonprescription Drugs and Dietary Supplements, 2000, 21st ed. Medical Economics, 2000.

Quick Look Drug Book, 2001. J. B. Lippincott, 2001.

General Medicine

Merck Manual, Diagnosis and Therapy, 17th ed. Merck Publishing Group, Inc., 1999.

Grammar Review/Style Manuals

Fordney, Marilyn T., March O. Diehl, and Maureen Pfeiffer. *Medical Transcription Guide: Do's and Dont's*, 2nd ed. W. B. Saunders Company, 1999.

Mitchell, Carol A. *Machine Transcription*, 4th ed. Glencoe McGraw-Hill, 2001.

Sabin, William A. *The Gregg Reference Manual*, 9th ed. Glencoe McGraw-Hill, 2001.

Tessier, Claudia. *The AAMT Book of Style for Medical Transcription*. American Association for Medical Transcription, 1995.

Web Sites

Web sites change often, particularly drug indexes. Please use the search engine to determine new sites.

AltaVista.com (search engine)

Healthatoz.com (search engine)

healthinfoseek.com

mwsearch.com (search engine)

intelihealth.com

medterms.com

merck.com/pubs/mmanual

mtdesk.com

pharminfo.com (drug index)

Rxlist.com (drug index)

spellex.com/speller.htm

Appendix F: AAMT Job Description

The American Association for Medical Transcription (AAMT) represents the medical transcription profession. AAMT has created a model job description, which is a practical useful compilation of the basic job responsibilities of a medical transcriptionist.

AAMT defines a medical transcriptionist as a medical language specialist who interprets and transcribes dictation by physicians and other health care professionals regarding patient assessment, workup, therapeutic procedures, clinical course, diagnosis, prognosis, etc., in order to document patient care and facilitate delivery of health care services.

AAMT Model Job Description

Knowledge, Skills, and Abilities

1. Minimum education level of associate degree or its equivalent in work experience and continuing education.
2. Knowledge of medical terminology, anatomy and physiology, clinical medicine, surgery, diagnostic tests, radiology, pathology, pharmacology, and the various medical specialties as required in areas of responsibility.
3. Knowledge of medical transcription guidelines and practices.
4. Excellent written and oral communication skills, including English usage, grammar, punctuation and style.
5. Ability to understand diverse accents and dialects and varying dictation styles.
6. Ability to use designated reference materials.
7. Ability to operate designated word processing, dictation, and transcription equipment, and other equipment as specified.
8. Ability to work independently with minimal supervision.
9. Ability to work under pressure with time constraints.
10. Ability to concentrate.
11. Excellent listening skills.
12. Excellent eye, hand, and auditory coordination.
13. Certified medical transcriptionist (CMT) status preferred.

Working Conditions

General office environment. Quiet surroundings. Adequate lighting.

Physical Demands

Primarily sedentary work with continuous use of earphones, keyboard, foot control, and, where applicable, video display terminal.

Job Responsibilities

1. Transcribes medical dictation to provide a permanent record of patient care.

2. Demonstrates an understanding of the medicolegal implications and responsibilities related to the transcription of patient records to protect the patient and the business/institution.

3. Operates designated word processing, dictation, and transcription equipment as directed to complete assignments.

4. Follows policies and procedures to contribute to the efficiency of the medical transcription department.

5. Expands job-related knowledge and skills to improve performance and adjust to change.

6. Uses interpersonal skills effectively to build and maintain cooperative working relationships.

Performance Standards

1.1 Applies knowledge of medical terminology, anatomy and physiology, and English language rules to the transcription and proofreading of medical dictation from originators with various accents, dialects, and dictation styles.

1.2 Recognizes, interprets, and evaluates inconsistencies, discrepancies, and inaccuracies in medical dictation, and appropriately edits, revises, and clarifies them without altering the meaning of the dictation or changing the dictator's style.

1.3 Clarifies dictation that is unclear or incomplete, seeking assistance as necessary.

1.4 Flags reports requiring the attention of the supervisor or dictator.

1.5 Uses reference materials appropriately and efficiently to facilitate the accuracy, clarity, and completeness of reports.

1.6 Meets quality and productivity standards and deadlines established by employer.

1.7 Verifies patient information for accuracy and completeness.

1.8 Formats reports according to established guidelines.

2.1 Understands and complies with policies and procedures related to medicolegal matters, including confidentiality, amendment of medical records, release of information, patients' rights, medical records as legal evidence, informed consent, etc.

2.2 Meets standards of professional and ethical conduct.

2.3 Recognizes and reports unusual circumstances and/or information with possible risk factors to appropriate risk management personnel.

2.4 Recognizes and reports problems, errors, and discrepancies in dictation and patient records to appropriate manager.

2.5 Consults appropriate personnel regarding dictation that may be regarded as unprofessional, frivolous, insulting, inflammatory, or inappropriate.

3.1 Uses designated equipment effectively, skillfully, and efficiently.

3.2 Maintains equipment and work area as directed.

3.3 Assesses condition of equipment and furnishings, and reports need for replacement or repair.

4.1 Demonstrates an understanding of policies, procedures, and priorities, seeking clarification as needed.

4.2 Reports to work on time, as scheduled, and is dependable and cooperative.

4.3 Organizes and prioritizes assigned work, and schedules time to accommodate work demands, turnaround-time requirements, and commitments.

4.4 Maintains required records, providing reports as scheduled and upon request.

4.5 Participates in quality assurance programs.

4.6 Participates in evaluation and selection of equipment and furnishings.

4.7 Provides administrative/clerical/technical support as needed and as assigned.

5.1 Participates in in-service and continuing education activities.

5.2 Provides documentation of in-service and continuing education activities.

5.3 Reviews trends and developments in medicine, English usage, technology, and transcription practices, and shares knowledge with colleagues.

5.4 Documents new and revised terminology, definitions, styles, and practices for reference and application.

5.5 Participates in the evaluation and selection of books, publications, and other reference materials.

6.1 Works and communicates in a positive and cooperative manner with management and supervisory staff, medical staff, co-workers and other health care personnel, and with patients and their families when providing information and services, seeking assistance and clarification, and resolving problems.

6.2 Contributes to team efforts.

6.3 Carries out assignments responsibly.

6.4 Participates in a positive and cooperative manner during staff meetings.

6.5 Handles difficult and sensitive situations tactfully.

6.6 Responds well to supervision.

6.7 Shares information with co-workers.

6.8 Assists with training of new employees as needed.

Glossary

A	abduction	moves away from the body
	abrasion	removal of superficial layer of skin
	abscess	localized collection of pus
	ache	pain that persists
	acne	inflammation of sebaceous glands
	acute	having a short and sharp course
	adduction	moves toward the midline of the body
	adenopathy	enlargement of lymph nodes (also called *lymphadenopathy*)
	adolescent	person in the teen years
	afebrile	not having an elevated body temperature
	aggravating	make worse
	AIDS	acquired immunodeficiency syndrome
	alcoholism	chronic, excessive drinking of alcohol
	alignment	proper position
	allergy	sensitivity to a substance that results in symptoms
	ambulate	to walk about
	anemia	low hemoglobin
	angina	constricting chest pain
	anomaly	abormality; deviation from normal
	anorexia	diminished appetite
	anterior/ventral	toward the front
	anuria	absence of urine
	aphasia	impaired speech
	appendicitis	inflammation of appendix
	apraxia	inability to perform voluntary movement
	arteriosclerotic heart disease (ASHD)	hardening of the coronary arteries
	arthritis	joint inflammation
	asepsis	cleanliness
	asthma	condition of lungs causing difficulty breathing
	astigmatism	warped or distorted image
	ataxia	inability to control voluntary muscles for movement
	atrophy	wasting of a structure
	audible	to be heard
	avulsion	separation
	axillary	pertaining to the armpit
B	bacteriuria	bacteria in urine
	barrel chested	having a rounded (barrel or box car) shape to chest
	basal cell carcinoma	skin cancer
	belch	burp
	benign	of mild character
	benign prostatic hypertrophy (BPH)	overgrowth of prostatic tissue (not malignant)
	blepharitis	inflammation of the eyelid
	blister	fluid-filled structure under the skin
	boil	infection in a hair follicle
	bradycardia	slow pulse

Glossary

	breadth	width
	breech	buttocks presenting at vaginal opening at time of delivery
	bronchitis	inflammation in the bronchi
	bronchospasm	contraction of bronchi, causing narrowing of the lumen (opening)
	bruit	murmur
	bulging	swelling
	bursitis	inflammation of bursa
C	calcification	deposit of lime or calcium salt
	calculus (plural, calculi)	stone
	cancer	malignant growth
	carpal tunnel syndrome	wrist pain and weakness due to pressure on median nerve
	cataract	loss of transparency of eye lens
	catheter	tubular instrument to allow passage of air or fluid
	cellulitis	inflammation of skin and subcutaneous tissue
	cephalopelvic	disproportional size of fetal head to maternal pelvis
	cerebral palsy	spasms or paralysis due to brain lesion, usually suffered at birth
	cerebrovascular accident	stroke
	cervicitis	inflammation of mucosa of the cervix
	Chlamydia	type of venereal disease
	cholecystitis	inflammation of gallbladder
	cholelithiasis	stones in the gallbladder
	chronic obstructive pulmonary disease (COPD)	diseases in which forced expiratory flow is slowed
	chronic	marked by slow progress and long continuance
	circumduction (of the shoulders and hips)	allows movement in a circle
	cirrhosis	progressive liver disease
	claustrophobia	morbid fear of confinement
	clay-colored stool	no color to the stools
	clubbing	abnormality of fingertips indicative of chronic lung disease
	colic	sharp, spasmodic abdominal pain
	Colles fracture	fractured radius with displacement
	comedos	blackheads caused by plugged oil gland
	concussion	violent jarring of brain
	configuration	arrangement or form
	congenital	existing at birth
	congestion	accumulation of abnormal amount of fluid or blood
	congestive heart failure (CHF)	increased fluid, especially in lungs, due to poor circulation
	conjunctivitis	inflammation of conjunctiva
	consolidation	condition of becoming solid

	constipation	infrequent hard, dry stool
	constriction	tightening, squeezing, contracting, or narrowing
	contaminate	to render unclean
	contraindication	inadvisable
	contusion	bruise
	convulsion	seizure
	copious	large amount
	coronary artery disease	disease affecting blood vessels that supply heart muscle
	costochondritis	inflammation of cartilage between ribs
	cough	sudden forcing of air from respiratory tract
	crackle	sound in lungs similar to rolling hairs between fingers
	crepitus	crackling or bubbling sound or feeling
	crisis	a sudden change
	croup	noisy, barklike respirations
	cyanosis	bluish tinge to skin due to circulatory or respiratory problems
	cyst	sac containing fluid
	cystic breast disease	formation of fluid or semisolid sac of breast tissue
	cystitis	inflammation of the bladder
	cystocele	herniation of bladder into vaginal wall
D	debris	material that does not belong in that area
	deep venous thrombosis (DVT)	formation of blood clots in veins
	degenerative arthritis	deterioration of joint structures
	degenerative disk disease (DDD)	deterioration of disk
	degenerative joint disease (DJD)	deterioration of joints
	dehydration	reduction of water content
	dermatitis	general term indicating inflammation of skin
	detached retina	retina pulled away from the choroid
	diabetes mellitus	inadequate glucose metabolism (type I, juvenile onset; type II, adult onset; gestational, pregnancy related)
	diaphoresis	perspiration; sweating
	diarrhea	frequent watery or nonformed stool
	dilate	to widen
	disease	illness
	dislocation	displacement; disruption of proper position
	disposition	treatment or management
	distal	away from point of origin
	distention	state of being stretched or distended
	diverticulitis	inflammation of a diverticulum
	dribbling	falling in drops involuntarily
	dysmenorrhea	menstrual cramps
	dyspepsia	indigestion

	dysphagia	difficulty swallowing
	dysplasia	abnormal tissue development
	dyspnea	difficulty breathing
	dysrhythmia	abnormal heart rhythm; arrhythmia
	dysuria	difficult or painful urination
E	ecchymosis	black and blue or purple discoloration of skin caused by bruise
	eclampsia	toxic condition of pregnancy
	ectopic	misplaced
	edema	accumulation of excess fluid in the tissue
	effusion	excessive fluid in joint space
	elicit	reveal; provide
	emesis	vomiting
	emphysema	abnormal increase in size of air sacs (alveoli)
	endometriosis	formation of endometrial tissue in the pelvic cavity outside the uterus
	epididymitis	inflammation of epididymis
	epilepsy	excessive electrical activity in the brain
	epistaxis	nosebleed
	erosion	wearing away
	eruption	rash
	erythema	reddish color to skin
	etiology	study of cause of disease
	euthyroid	normally functioning thyroid gland
	eversion	turning outward
	exacerbation	increase in symptom(s)
	excoriation	break in skin caused by surface trauma; scratch
	exophthalmos (exophthalmus)	bulging eyes
	extension	increases the size of an angle
	exudate	material deposited on tissue as a result of infection
F	fatigue	feeling of tiredness
	fetal heart tones (FHT)	pulse rate of fetus
	fibrotic	referring to tough or strong material
	fingerbreadths	width of a finger; almost an inch
	fissure	furrow; crack
	flank	region between ribs and hip
	flatulence/flatus	excessive gas in GI tract
	flexion	decreases the size of an angle
	fluctuant	wavelike motion
	fracture	break
	frequency	something that happens at short intervals, as urination
	friction rub	grating or creaking sound when pleurae rub together
G	gait	method of walking
	gallop	fast triple rhythm of heartbeat
	gastritis	inflammation of stomach

	gastroenteritis	inflammation of stomach and intestine
	gaunt	thin and bony; emaciated
	gaze	look steadily
	gestation	pregnancy
	glaucoma	disease characterized by increased intraocular pressure
	glomerulonephritis	inflammation of the filtering mechanism within kidney
	glycosuria	glucose (sugar) in the urine
	goiter	enlargement of thyroid gland
	gonorrhea (GC)	type of venereal disease
	gouty arthritis	deposits of crystals in joints
	Graves' disease	overactive thyroid characterized by toxic goiter
	gravid	pregnant
	gravida	pregnant woman
H	hematemesis	vomiting blood
	hematochezia	bloody stools
	hematuria	blood in urine
	hemorrhage	bleeding not easily stopped; excessive bleeding
	hemorrhoids	dilated vein in rectal area
	hepatitis	inflammation of liver
	hernia	protrusion of an organ
	herniated disk	disk that protrudes
	herpes	eruption of vesicles on reddish bases caused by a virus
	hesitancy	involuntary delay in starting the urinary stream
	hiatal hernia	protrusion of part of stomach through diaphragm
	hoarse	having a rough, harsh voice
	horizontal/transverse	across
	human Papilloma virus (HPV)	type of venereal disease
	hydration	adequate tissue fluid; not dehydrated
	hydronephrosis	dilation of kidneys due to obstruction in flow of urine
	hypercholesterolemia	increased amount of cholesterol (fatty substances) in the blood
	hyperglycemia	too much glucose in the blood; high blood sugar
	hypertension	high blood pressure
	hyperthyroidism	excessive functioning activity of the thyroid
	hypertrophy	increase in size of an organ
	hypoglycemia	too little glucose in blood; low blood sugar
	hypokalemia	decreased potassium in blood
	hypothyroidism	deficiency of thyroid function

I

icterus	jaundice; yellowish color to skin or eyes
ileus	bowel obstruction
immobile	not capable of moving
impetigo	contagious superficial infection with vesicles and yellowish crusting
impingement	beyond the usual limit or location
incarceration	being trapped
incontinence	inability to control urination
indurated	hardened or firm
infection	invasion of area with pathogenic microorganisms
inferior	below
infiltrate	accumulation of fluid
inflammation	tissue reaction to injury (pain, warmth, swelling, redness)
inguinal hernia	hernia located in the groin
injection	congestion or increase in fluid
injury	damage; trauma
introitus	entrance
inversion	turns inward
ischemia	decreased blood supply

K

keloid	overgrowth of scar tissue

L

labyrinthitis	inflammation in inner ear
laceration	accidental tear of skin
lateral	side
lesion	injury or pathological change in tissue
lethargy	unconsciousness from which one can be aroused, but not without relapses
lightheadedness	dizziness
low-grade fever	mildly elevated temperature

M

maculae	colored spots on skin
macular degeneration	deterioration of retina
malaise	feeling of uneasiness; of being "out-of-sorts" feeling
malignant	harmful; causing death
manual	pertaining to the hand
mastalgia	breast pain
medial	middle
melena	dark, tarry stools
menopause	cessation of menses
menorrhagia	excessive bleeding at time of period
menses	menstrual period
metastasis	spread of disease to another body part
metrorrhagia	bleeding between periods
migraine	severe headache
modalities	form, method
mononucleosis	abnormally large number of leukocytes in blood
multiple sclerosis	brain or spinal cord plaque causing tremor, paralysis, or disturbed speech

murmur	abnormal heart sound coming from heart valves
myocardial infarction (MI)	inadequate blood supply to heart muscle; heart attack
myositis	inflammation of muscle

N

nausea	feeling of having to vomit
necrosis	dead tissue; not viable
neonatal	birth to 28 days
nephrolithiasis	the condition of having a kidney stone
nephropathy	kidney disease
neuropathy	disease involving nerves
nevus	circumscribed, pigmented (shade of brown) area of skin; mole
nocturia	urination at night
nodule	knob, mass, or swelling
nonunion	unhealed fracture site
normocephalic	normal-sized head
nuchal rigidity	stiff neck
numbness	absence of feeling
nystagmus	jerking eye movement

O

obese	excessively fat
obstruction	blockage
occlusion	closed
occult	hidden
oligomenorrhea	scanty menstruation
oliguria	scanty urination
orchitis	inflammation of the testis
orthopnea	breathing discomfort when lying flat
osteoporosis	reduction in bone density
otitis media	inflammation of middle ear

P

palpitation	patient's awareness of heartbeat
pancreatitis	inflammation of pancreas
papule	pimple
paralysis	loss of voluntary movement
paresthesia	abnormal sensation; tingling
Parkinson's disease	shaking or trembling palsy
paronychia	inflammation of the nail fold
parous	having given birth
paroxysm	spasm; sudden recurrence
partum	delivery of fetus
patent	open
pediculosis	lice
pelvic inflammatory disease (PID)	inflammation of uterus, tubes, and ovaries
pendulous	hanging freely
peripheral	near the outside; away from heart
pharyngitis	inflammation of pharynx (throat)
phlegm	abnormal amounts of sticky mucus in the mouth and the throat
photophobia	sensitivity to light
plantar wart	wart on sole of foot

pneumonia	inflammation of lung tissue
polydipsia	increased thirst
polyp	projecting tissue mass
polyphagia	increased appetite
polyuria	excessive urination
posterior/dorsal	toward the back
postural	pertaining to position or posture
premenstrual syndrome (PMS)	group of symptoms occurring before the menstrual period
presents	appear for examination
prognosis	the outcome
prolapse of uterus	displacement of uterus into vagina
pronation (of the forearm)	places the palm down
prophylaxis	prevention
prosthesis	artificial substitute for missing part
proteinuria	protein in urine
provisional	temporary
proximal	nearer to point of origin
pruritus	itching
ptosis	downward organ displacement
punctate	tiny specks
purulent	containing pus
pustule	pimple with pus
pyelonephritis	inflammation of kidney
pyuria	pus in urine

Q

quadrant	quarter of a section

R

radiate	to spread
radiculopathy	disease of spinal nerve roots
rales	rattle heard on auscultation of chest
rectocele	herniation of rectum into vaginal wall
recumbent	lying down, reclining
recur	to happen again
reflux	backward flow
regimen	program or plan
residual urine	urine left in bladder after urination
retention	keeping in
rheumatoid arthritis	joint inflammation with constitutional symptoms
rhinitis	inflammation of the nasal mucosa
rhinorrhea	runny nose
rhonchi	musical pitch heard on auscultation of chest
rotation	moves the head from side to side
rub	abnormal heart sound (grating or scratchy)
ruga (rugae)	fold, ridge

S

scabies	itching eruption caused by mite
sciatica	pain in lower back and hip radiating down posterior thigh
seborrhea	overproduction of sebum from sebaceous glands, producing oily skin

sensitivity	responding to
septic	not clean; contaminated
sexually transmitted diseases (STDs)	venereal disease
shotty nodes	BB-like (very tiny bumps) feeling of lymph nodes
sibling	offspring of the same parents
sickle cell anemia	inherited abnormality of erythrocytes
sinusitis	inflammation of the sinuses
specimen	sample
sprain	twisting-type injury
sputum	material raised from the lungs
stasis ulcer	ulcer due to poor blood flow
stat	right now
status post	condition that has occurred
stenosis	narrowing
sterile	free of all microorganisms and spores
strain	muscle injury caused by overuse or improper use
strangulation	constriction of blood flow
stress incontinence	involuntarily expelling of urine during coughing, sneezing, laughing, etc.
stricture	narrowing of hollow structure
sty; stye	inflammation of oil gland of eyelid
sublingual	under the tongue
suboptimal	less than desired
superior	above
supination (of the forearm)	places the palm up
supple	easily moveable
suppurative	forming pus (purulent material)
suture	noun: threadlike material, stitch; verb: to sew or stitch
symmetric	equal
symptom	sign
syncope	fainting
syndrome	group of signs or symptoms

T

tachycardia	rapid heartbeat
tachypnea	increased rate of breathing
tendonitis or tendinitis	inflammation of tendon
therapy	treatment
thrombophlebitis	inflammation of vein due to blood clot
thrombosis	blood clot
thrush	fungal or yeast infection of mouth tissue, often after treatment with antibiotics
thyrotoxicosis	extremely overactive thyroid gland
tonsillitis	inflammation of the tonsils
tract	pathway
transient ischemic attack (TIA)	short-term interruption of blood supply to brain
trauma	injury
tremulous	quivering
Trichomonas	parasitic infection

U

ulcer	open sore
upper respiratory tract infection (URI)	infection of upper air passages, not involving the lungs
ureteritis	inflammation of ureter
ureterolithiasis	stone in ureter
urethritis	inflammation of urethra
urgency	desire to void immediately
urinary tract infection (UTI)	infection of urinary tract, not including kidneys

V

vaginosis	bacterial infection of vagina
varicose veins	enlarged, tortuous vessels
vascular insufficiency	inadequate blood vessels
verruca	overgrowth of dermis, caused by virus; wart
vertex	top of the skull
vertical	up and down
vertigo	dizziness
vesicle	circumscribed elevation of skin containing fluid

W

wheeze	whistling or squeaking sound when breathing
whiplash	neck injury when struck from behind
wrinkle	fold, crease

Index

Index

Cecum, 87, 88
Ceftin, 60
-cele, 14
-centesis, 14
Central nervous system (CNS), 164–166
Cerebellum, 164, 165
Cerebrospinal fluid (CSF), 165
Cerebrum, 164, 165
Certified medical transcriptionist (CMT), 7
Cerumen, 56, 168
Cervical os, 131
Cervical region, 55
Cervix, 131
Cesarean section (C-section), 135, 138
Chart Note (model), 21, 23
Charts. *See* Patient medical records (PMR)
Chest, 54
Chest x-rays, 59
Chief complaint (CC), 18
Chlamydia, 134
Chlorides, 74, 90
Chlorpheniramine, 92
Cholecystectomy, 91
Cholesterol, 74, 90
chord, cord, 173
Choroid, 167, 168
Circumcision, 135
Circumduction, 15, 16
Clean-catch/midstream, 117
Clinical data, 16–17
Clitoris, 131
Closed reduction, 153
coarse, course, 61
Code of ethics, 5–6
Colon, 86–87, 91
Colonoscopy, 91
Colons (:), 108
Color
    of skin, 41
    of urine, 117
Commas (,)
    with equal adjectives, 29
    with independent clauses, 156
    with introductory clauses and phrases, 46
Compazine, 119
Complete blood count (CBC), 74, 90
Compound nouns, 156
Computed tomography (CT) scans, 163, 171
Conclusion, on medical record, 18
Condyle, 147
Conjunctiva, 167, 168
continual, continuous, 108

contra-, 14
Cornea, 167, 168
Coronary artery bypass graft (CABG), 75
Cortex, 115
Costovertebral angle (CVA), 114
Coumadin, 44, 76
course, coarse, 61
Cranial nerves, 166, 167
Creatinine, 74, 90, 117
Crutch, 153
Cryosurgery, 43
Cryotherapy, 135
C-section (cesarean section), 138
CT scans, 163, 171
Cul-de-sac, 131
Culture, 59
Cutaneous layer, 40
Cystorrhaphy, 135
Cystoscopy, 119

D

Daypro, 154
Debridement, 43
Deep tendon reflexes (DTRs), 151, 169
Demerol, 76
Dentistry, 3
Dermatology, 3
Dermis, 40
Descending colon, 87, 88
Diabetes mellitus, adult onset (type II), 104
Diagnosis, on medical record, 18
Dialysis, 119
Diaphragm, 54
Diastole, 71, 72–73
Differential, 74
Digestion, 86
Digestive system, 85–94
Digital dictation systems, 7
Digoxin (Lanoxin), 76
Dilatation & curettage (D&C), 135
Dilation/dilatation, 119
Directional terms, 14–15
discreet, discrete, 78
Disposition, in patient medical records, 18
Distal, 15
Doppler ultrasound, 75
Dorsal, 14
Dorsalis pedis, 72
Doxycycline, 135
Duodenum, 86, 88
Duoderm, 106
Dura mater, 166
dys-, 14

E

E. coli (Escherichia coli), 118
Eardrums, 168
Earphones, 7
Ears, 56, 168
ECG, EKG, 69, 75
-ectomy, 14
Edema, 73
EEG (electroencephalogram), 171
E.E.S. (brand of erythromycin), 44
effect, affect, 29
Elasticity, 41
Electrocardiogram (ECG), 69, 75
Electroencephalogram (EEG), 171
Electrolytes, 74, 90
Electromyogram (EMG), 153
Elimination, 40, 86
Emergency medicine, 3
EMG (electromyogram), 153
-emia, 14
Enalapril, 76
endo-, 14
Endocardium, 71
Endocrine system, 101–108
Endocrinology, 3
Endodontist, 3
Endometrial lining, 131
Endometrium, 131
Endoscopy, 91
Eosinophils, 70
epi-, 14
Epidermis, 40
Epididymus, 130
Epiglottis, 55
Epigrastrium, 87
Epiphysis, 147
Epithelial tissue, 40
erythmia, arythmia, 78
Erythrocytes (red blood cells), 70
Erythromycin, 44
Esophagus, 86, 88
Estraderm, 106, 135
Estrogen, 131
Ethical codes, 5–6
Eustachian tubes, 168, 169
Eversion, 15, 16
ex-, 14
Examination methods, 17
excess, access, assess, 29
Excision, 43
Excretion, 70
Expander software, 9
Expiration, 54
Extension, 15, 16
External genitalia, 130
Extraocular movements or motions (EOMs), 169
Extraocular muscles (EOMs), 167
Eyes, 56, 167

Index

Index

Index

Index

S

sac, sack, 108
Saline, 44
Salivary glands, 87, 88
Saphenous vein, 72
Sciatic notch, 147
Sclera, 167, 168
-scopy, 14
Scrotum, 130
Sebaceous (oil/sebum) glands, 40
self-, hyphenation with, 62
Semen, 130
semi-, 14
Semicolons (;), 108
Semilunar, 71
Seminal vesicles, 130
Sensation, 40
Sense organs, 167–169
Sensory nerves, 164
Septra, Septra DS (double strength), 119
Shaft, 147
sight, site, 45
Sigmoid, 87
Signs, 151
Sinoatrial (SA) node, 72
Sinus, 147
Sinus films, 59
site, sight, 45
Sitz bath, 135
Skene's glands, 131
Skin, 39–46
Sling, 153
SOAP method, 21
soar, sore, 45
Social history (SH), 18
Sodium, 74, 90
Sodium Sulamyd, 172
Soft palate, 55
sore, soar, 45
Specialties and subspecialties, 2, 3–4
Specific gravity, 117
Speculum, 132
Speech recognition systems, 8–9
Spelling checkers, 8
Sperm, 130
Spermatic cord, 130
Spinal cord, 165, 166
Spinal nerves, 166, 167
Spirometry, 60
Spleen, 71, 88
Splint, 153
Sternum, 132
Stomach, 86, 88
-stomy, 14
Stool, 88

Stress (exercise) ECG, 75
Styloid, 147
sub-, 14
Subarachnoid space, 166
Subclavian artery, 72
Subcutaneous tissue, 40
Subjective (S) findings, 21
Submandibular, 55
Subscripts, 90
Suffixes, 14
Sulfacetamide, 172
super-, 14
Superior, 15
Superior vena cava, 71, 72
Supination, 15, 16
supra-, 14
Suprapubic, 114
Suspected, 18
Sweat glands, 40
Symmetric, 15
Synovial fluid, 146
Synthroid, 106
Systole, 71, 72–73

T

T3, 106
T-4, 106
Tactile sensation, 169
Tagamet, 92
Tamoxifen, 135
Tear glands, 167, 168
Teeth, 88
Temperature, skin, 41
Tendons, 146
Terminology, 14–16
    directional, 14–15
    movement types, 15–16
    prefixes, 14
    suffixes, 14
Testes, 102, 103, 130
Testicular self-exam, 135
Testosterone, 130
Tetanus booster, 44
Texture, skin, 41
than, then, 93
Thoracic surgery, 4
Thrombocytes, 70
Thyroid gland, 102, 103, 104
Thyroid scan, 106
Thyroidectomy, 106
Tibial artery and vein, 72
Time, units of, 46
Titles, abbreviating, 46
-tomy, 14
Tongue, 88
Tonsillectomy and adenoidectomy (T&A), 60

Tonsils, 49, 55, 56, 60
Toradol, 92
TPAL terminology, 138
Trachea, 54, 55
trans-, 14
Transcription guidelines, 9
Transcription process, 7–9
    dictation systems, 7
    speech recognition systems, 8–9
Transurethral resection of prostate (TUR; TURP), 119
Transverse, 14
Transverse colon, 87, 88
Treadmill exercise, 75
Treatment, in patient medical records, 18
Triamcinolone (Aristospan), 154
Trichomonas and yeast (T&Y), 134
Tricuspid valve, 72
Triglycerides, 90
-tripsy, 14
Trochanter, 147
-trophy, 14
TSH, 106
Tuberosity, 147
Turbinates, 54
Turgor, skin, 41
24-hour urinalysis, 117
Tylenol, 60
Tylenol #3, 44
Tympanic membranes (TMs), 56, 168, 169
Tympanogram, 171
Type I diabetes, 104
Type II diabetes, 104
Types of movement, 15–16

U

Ultralente insulin injections, 107
Ultrasound, 91, 118, 134
Upper gastrointestinal (GI) series, 85, 91
Upper GI tract, 87
Ureterovesical junction, 114
Ureters, 114, 115
Urethra, 114, 115, 130
Urethral glands, 131
Uric acid, 152
Urinalysis (UA), 117–118
Urinary system, 113–121
Urine, 114
Urine culture (UC) and sensitivity, 117
Urology, 4
Uterine suspension, 135

Index

V

Vagina, 131
Valium, 172
Valves, heart, 70, 71, 72
Vaporizer, 60
Vas deferens, 130
Vasectomy, 135
Veins, 71, 72
Ventolin (albuterol), 60
Ventral, 14
Ventriculogram, 75
Vertebra, 165
Vertical, 14
Visine, 172
Vistaril, 76
Visual refraction, 171
Vitamins, 86
Void, 114
Voiding cystourethrogram (VCUG), 113, 118
Vulva, 131

W

Water, 86
WBC, wbc, 59, 118
White blood cell count (WBC), 74, 118
White blood cells (wbc; leukocytes), 70

X

x-ray, 59
X-Ray Report (model), 25
Xylocaine (lidocaine), 44, 76

Z

Zantac, 92
Zoloft, 106